THE

THE COMPLETE

ANTENATAL

GUIDE TO

TESTING

TESTING IN

HANDBOOK

PREGNANCY

VIVIENNE PARRY

PAN BOOKS

London, Sydney and Auckland

First published 1993 by Pan Books Ltd

a division of Pan Macmillan Publishers Limited
Cavaye Place London SW10 9PG
and Basingstoke

Associated companies throughout the world

ISBN 0 330 32852 2

9 8 7 6 5 4 3 2 1

A CIP catalogue record for this book is available from
the British Library

Typeset by Cambridge Composing (UK) Limited,
Cambridge
Printed and bound in Great Britain by
Cox & Wyman Limited, Reading

Contents

Acknowledgements

The author and publishers gratefully acknowledge the following for permission to quote:

An Introduction to Medical Genetics Eighth Edition, J. A. Fraser Roberts and M. E. Pembrey, Oxford University Press, 1985
ABC of Clinical Genetics, Helen M. Kingston, British Medical Journal, 1990
Biology A Functional Approach Third Edition, M. B. V. Roberts, Thomas Nelson & Sons Ltd, 1982
Antenatal Diagnosis of Foetal Abnormalities, eds J. O. Drife and D. Donnai, Springer Verlag, 1991
Introduction to Animal Parasitology Second Edition, J. D. Smyth, Hodder & Stoughton, 1976
British Medical Journal Volume 305, Dr Susan M. Hall, 1992
Antenatal and Neonatal Screening, Ed N. Wald, Oxford University Press, 1984

Foreword

The vast majority of babies are born normal. However, 3–5 per cent are born with some form of handicapping condition. These abnormalities usually arise out of the blue, with no previous family history of handicap. It is for this reason that a series of screening tests is undertaken during the course of pregnancy to identify women at higher or lower risk for a given abnormality. Major medical advances over the last few years have made it possible to reassure most parents that their baby is healthy. For those few parents whose baby has an abnormality, the various tests can provide information on the possible severity of the condition, and help them decide on the subsequent course of their pregnancy.

Every year in Britain alone, close to a million pregnant women are confronted by a rapidly increasing number of options for antenatal testing. This book explains how abnormalities arise, how the various screening and diagnostic tests are carried out, their risks, and the information they provide.

Vivienne Parry is a great communicator. Through her work at Birthright, the mother and baby research charity of the Royal College of Obstetricians and Gynaecologists, she knows the concerns of pregnant women. Her background as a scientist, journalist and mother has enabled her to write a book which, despite its serious nature, is easy to read, witty and highly informative.

Kypros Nicolaides
Professor of Fetal Medicine
King's College Hospital, London

Introduction

WHAT ARE TESTS FOR?

Pregnancy is beset with uncertainty. There are very few women who can, with hand on heart, say that right from the moment they discovered they were pregnant, they felt sure that in the fullness of time they would be holding a healthy baby in their arms. This feeling of uncertainty has, if anything, increased over the past few years. As more and more antenatal tests become available we have become less and less sure about our ability to have a healthy baby.

When we think about testing in pregnancy, we are very much influenced by our own experience of handicap and disability. For those with genetic disease in the family testing is a modern miracle, giving the chance of a healthy family to a couple who have the dark spectre of genetic disease hanging over them. To others, testing is seen as conferring some sort of guarantee of health on their baby. Yet another group of women would rather not have testing at all, preferring instead to learn about their baby when it's born. And there are many more women who are confused about what is available, what the tests are for, and what the risks of handicap are, anyway.

Testing is an immensely personal decision which is explored in greater depth in Chapter 2. It is a complex issue that is made immeasurably harder by lack of information. The aim then, in writing this book, is not to give you advice about what you should do, or even tell you whether you should opt for testing in the first place. It is simply to provide you with a starting block of knowledge on which to base your decisions.

It has been hard to write a book like this without using the words 'abnormal' or 'handicapped'. They are not words that I particularly like, but they are the words that are most commonly used and understood. Babies born with diseases such as spina bifida are different. Their 'handicap' is created by the very fact that they are different and by the way that society treats them. Having a baby that is different has enormous implications. It poses questions that we may not want to face, like 'Could I manage?', or 'Could I cope with my child being different?'. Very often we have not resolved these questions in our minds when we embark on testing, preferring instead to think that we will cross this bridge if or when we come to it.

The first question you may want to ask is, how likely am I to have a baby with a handicap? There is a common assumption that if there is no history of handicap in the family, then your baby is not at risk. In fact, it is estimated that half the world's women will conceive a pregnancy with a chromosome abnormality. Most such pregnancies end in miscarriage, sometimes before the woman is even aware that she is pregnant. Of approximately 750,000 babies born in Britain each year, some 18–20,000 – that is 1 in 40 births – will have a disability. For the vast majority of parents (65 per cent) there was no prior history of handicap in the family.

In this introduction the various types of handicap are outlined, so as to make clear what the tests are for. In later chapters each test is explained in detail, while the directory at the end of the book describes the most common types of disease and handicap.

Some forms of handicap, such as spina bifida, are obvious almost immediately. Some, such as cystic fibrosis, may be symptomless at first and will be diagnosed only when the baby gets a bit older. Others such as haemophilia can't be seen, but are there none the less. Handicapping conditions can be grouped into three main types.

Physical Defects

Called congenital malformations – where congenital means simply present at birth – these form the largest group of handicaps. Table 1 lists the most common types, with heart defects being most frequent, followed by limb deformities and disorders of the central nervous system (such as spina bifida). Although some are inherited problems (as with some forms of heart defect) most come out of the blue, with no family history (something you will see described as 'sporadic'). Ultrasound is used to detect these sorts of physical handicaps.

Table 1: Approximate annual incidence of births of babies with congenital and genetically determined disorders in the UK (Total annual births about 700,000)

BABIES BORN WITH PHYSICAL MALFORMATIONS	
Inherited	1,400
Sporadic	10,500–14,000
INHERITED GENE DEFECTS	
e.g. cystic fibrosis, haemophilia	4,700–5,600
CHROMOSOME DISORDERS	
Inherited	420
Sporadic	1,800
Total	18,600–22,800

Physical abnormality may also be a pointer to disorders in the baby's genetic material, even though these can't in themselves be detected by ultrasound scanning. Finding that a baby has a heart defect should prompt another sort of testing, involving looking at a sample of the baby's cells, which might reveal, for instance, that the baby also has a chromosomal disorder such as Down's syndrome (50 per cent of Down's babies have associated heart problems). Alphafetoprotein (AFP) testing is another test for physical abnormality, where the presence of a specific chemical in the mother's blood may indicate the presence of one type of physical handicap, spina bifida, in the baby.

Inherited Genetic Disease

The next most common handicapping condition is inherited genetic disease. There is more about this on pages 10–18 but for the moment all you need to know is that every cell in our body contains a copy of a unique personal instruction manual. As with all manuals, a bit of gobbledegook arising as a result of a misprint may not matter, either because the sense of it remains the same, or because that bit of the manual wasn't very important. However, a one letter misprint could be crucial – such as an instruction in a manual that said 'Throw out the cat' instead of 'Throw out the mat'. It is these significant alterations to the manual, which are inherited by the baby, that cause genetic disease. It's called genetic because the manual is contained, as a sequence of chemical codes or genes, on microscopic paired structures called chromosomes which are found in each and every cell of the body. Overall, cystic fibrosis is the most common inherited genetic disease but in some ethnic groups other inherited genetic diseases may be much more important. For instance, the crippling blood disease sickle-cell anaemia is forty times more common than cystic fibrosis in communities of Afro-Caribbean origin.

Nearly 5,000 so-called single gene defects have been described to date, with more being added to the list all the time.

Chromosome Disorders

These are responsible for handicaps such as Down's syndrome and Turner's syndrome. In general these are not inherited conditions (although there are some which are). They arise because, either within the sperm or egg or at conception, chromosomes, while trying to sort themselves out properly, have got tangled up and haven't done what they should. Separating the chromosomes in a cell when it divides is a bit like having a great heap of green and white spaghetti on your plate and trying to sort it out into two piles, one green and one white. You'll find that bits of the green stick onto the white, some bits of spaghetti get broken, and some bits may disappear off the plate altogether during your sorting efforts. In general, chromosome disorders arise at conception, and will affect only that pregnancy. The point to remember about such disorders is that they were present right from the word go, and nothing that you did, or did not do, during your pregnancy could have caused them.

To detect both genetic disease and chromosome disorders in the baby, you need to obtain a sample of the baby's cells. These can be any sort of cells (remember, almost all cells in the baby's body contain the same set of chromosomal information, with a few well-known exceptions in the adult such as red blood cells). The most usual ways of obtaining these cells are either amniocentesis or chorionic villus sampling. Another way of obtaining this information is by looking at the chromosomes within the baby's white blood cells, and these are obtained by fetal blood sampling (most usually cordocentesis).

Recently, another method of detecting Down's syndrome has emerged. This involves looking at the levels of two chemicals in the mother's blood at a certain stage of pregnancy. This test, which may be combined with AFP determination, is called triple test and is discussed at greater length in Chapter 4.

One of the most important points to appreciate about antenatal diagnosis is that the tests are specific. You can only exclude that which you are specifically seeking to exclude. Although there is some overlap – physical markers pointing to genetic disease, for instance – if you are looking for genetic disease using amniocentesis, you may not find a physical handicap and vice versa. So, for example, if you are looking at a baby's karyotype (a spread of all the chromosomes in a cell), you can count the chromosomes to check that they are all there, you can look at their size and shape, you can look at the pattern of bands on them and in doing that, you will be able to come to the conclusion that this baby's chromosomes look normal. But you cannot possibly ask 5,000 questions of every sample of genetic material that you obtain in order to exclude all known single gene defects. All you can do is ask those questions which may be prompted by family history, such as 'Has this baby got muscular dystrophy?'.

But what makes genes go wrong? And how can you have a baby with a genetic problem when, as far as you know, you never had one? To understand this, you need to know something about the detail of chromosomes and the way that they carry genetic material.

CELLS AND CHROMOSOMES

When someone says to you, 'You look so like your mother', they are acknowledging something which has been known for thousands of years – that looks, height, hair colour, even body shape is passed on from parent to child. That both parents make a contribution is something that we can see for ourselves in the appearance of children whom we know – nose a bit like his dad, hair like his mum, and so on. The scientific study of the way that characteristics of the parents are inherited, both the things we can see and the things we can't, is called genetics. There has been an explosion of knowledge in this area recently, which is why you may be about to experience the dilemmas of testing but why your mother never even had to think about them. In fact, it wasn't until 1966 that the first antenatal diagnosis of Down's syndrome was made.

Each cell in your body, except sperm and eggs, carries an identical and absolutely unique instruction manual. This instruction manual dictates not only whether you are a man or a woman, whether your hair is red, your eyes green, but also carries information as to the precise structure and function of every bit of your body, right down to instructions for making tiny molecules of chemical that make individual cells work. This instruction manual is bequeathed to you by your parents, who each make an equal contribution to the contents of the manual, which is then duplicated again, and again, and again, so that every cell has the same manual.

The manual is, of course, rather more complex than I have made it appear here. For a start, it comes in 23 volumes. And there are two parts to each volume, one which came via your father and one via your mother. The two parts of the volume are about the same thing – you – but each part may carry different information about how a particular part of you should be put together. Sometimes this information can be conflicting and a choice must then be made between the two sets of instructions.

The instruction manual is summarized as a chemical code which rolls itself up into tightly coiled structures called chromosomes, which are present in every cell. The chromosomes can just be seen with the aid of a reasonably powerful microscope. In all the medical textbooks they are said to look like lamp brushes, whatever they are – fuzzy black bits is a more accurate description. The chromosomes hang about in pairs and there are 23 pairs altogether. Each pair is quite distinctive and each one has been given a number. Some pairs such as Chromosomes 1 and 2 are big, while others such as 20 and 21 are little. Twenty-two of the chromosome pairs are collectively called the autosomes, and the twenty-third pair

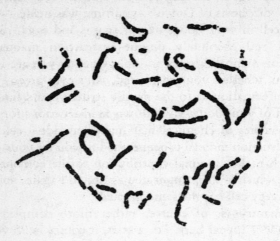

Figure 1a A karyotype and the chromosome spread from which it was constructed. The chromosomes are identified and put in this order by a cytologist to get a karyotype. Each chromosome can be identified with a microscope using special dyes or stains which give the characteristic pattern of alternating light and dark bands. (*From* An Introduction to Medical Genetics *Eighth Edition J. A. Fraser Roberts and M. E. Pembrey, Oxford University Press 1985*)

are the sex chromosomes that decide gender. So, if someone talks about a genetic disease that is autosomal, they mean one which is caused by an abnormality on one of the 22, and not on the sex chromosomes.

The chromosomes are each made of a single unbroken strand of a special material called DNA (deoxyribonucleic acid). DNA is not only capable of providing information in an easily deciphered form, but it is also able to reproduce itself – otherwise the information it contained couldn't be passed on to the next generation of cells.

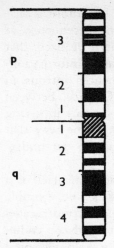

Figure 1b Simplified banding pattern of chromosome 1. The short arm of the chromosome is given the designation p, and the long arm, q. Each arm is subdivided numerically allowing precise localization of a structural abnormality. For instance, the gene linked to susceptibility to a type of kidney tumour called Wilm's tumour is 11p13 – meaning that it is on Chromosome No 11, on the short arm in position 13. (*From* ABC of Clinical Genetics *Helen M. Kingston, British Medical Journal 1990*)

Simplified banding pattern of chromosome 1.

DNA's structure is unique. Think of the DNA molecule as being like a piece of string on to which are threaded beads of four different colours, which are in reality four different amino acids (these are the body's chemical building blocks from which it manufactures many of the different chemicals that it requires). Three beads together constitute a codon. A sequence of codons, or sometimes even a single codon, is a gene. If you just have red (R), green (G), yellow (Y) and blue (B) beads to work from, there are 64 possible combinations of these beads. Each combination means something different, even though they are composed from the same beads – for instance RGY is different from YRG. More than this, if each little triplet of beads means something, then different combinations of triplets can be strung together, so that an infinitely variable set of sequences and instructions can be obtained.

The amount of information that the DNA molecule stores is absolutely vast – far more than we are ever likely to need.

Each chromosome contains 2–4,000 genes. As more is discovered about the human genome (the entire sequence of DNA in all the chromosomes), it has been realized that individual genes may contain both coding (information) sequences called exons, and non-coding sequences (introns) in their make-up and that there are tracts of 'space' between genes, called intergene segments, that play no part in giving information but are nevertheless important in the way that chapter headings and full stops are important to our understanding of a piece of writing.

The trick by which DNA manages to replicate itself is a stunning one but actually, like all the best tricks, very simple in concept. The DNA molecule is composed of two parallel strings of DNA, each with their attendant beads or codon which are fastened together and then wound in a double spiral way, the so-called 'double helix'. The two strings are able to unzip when it comes to cell replication time. One string, with its beads, then acts as a template for a new piece of DNA. Free beads (small molecules of amino acids) line up along the template, thus ensuring that the new bit of DNA is just like the old bit.

So that's the detail of genes, but how does it affect your baby?

Genetic Disease

We've said that the chromosomes are arranged in pairs and that they sometimes carry conflicting information at the same site or locus on each chromosome. These alternative forms of a gene or DNA sequence at the same site on a pair of chromosomes are called alleles (pronounced 'a-leels'). It's possible then to inherit a lethal gene from one parent, but for it to have no effect because the dominant information, the information selected as being right from the two bits contained on each of the two pairs of the chromosome, overrides it.

Almost all of us carry one or more inherited gene defect – for instance, 1 in 20 British people carry the cystic fibrosis gene. So, what we appear to be isn't necessarily what we are. What our genes say we are is called the genotype, and what we appear to be (our physical characteristics, right down to our blood groups) is called the phenotype.

Doctors often use a rather curious expression when talking about heredity – they talk about genes being 'expressed' or not. What they really mean is whether the effect of a particular gene is apparent in the phenotype, that is what a person appears to be, as well as in his genotype.

Hair colour is a good example of this because it is one of the rare characteristics that is controlled by a single gene pair. You may have genes that say both dark hair and red hair at the hair colour site on the relevant pair of chromosomes, but you will have – your genes will 'express' – brown hair, because your red hair gene is paired with a brown hair gene and the brown one is always dominant. The red hair colour gene is called a recessive gene. If both mother and father carry the gene for red hair (but have brown hair themselves), they will only have a red-haired child if the child inherits a double dose of the recessive red hair gene. Of course, hair colour has no medical significance, but many single gene defects are inherited in this so-called recessive way. Cystic fibrosis is the principal example and this explains why people who may have no family history of the disease have affected children. So long as they inherited a normal gene along with their CF gene, they will appear to be normal.

What, then, does carrying an autosomal recessive gene mean as far as your children are concerned? (Remember that autosomal just means hat the gene is on any of the chromosomes except the ones specifying sex.) As you will see, each of the children, no matter whether they are boys or girls, as in figure 2a, has a 1 in 4 chance of being affected and a 50:50 chance of being a carrier of the disease. The chances of being affected by

How Recessive inheritance works

Both parents, usually unaffected, carry a normal gene (**N**) which takes precedence over its faulty recessive counterpart (**r**).

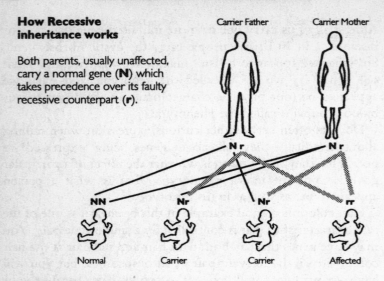

The odds for each child are:
1. a 25% risk of inheriting a 'double dose' of **r** genes which may cause a serious birth defect
2. a 25% chance of inheriting two **N**s, thus being unaffected
3. a 50% chance of being a carrier as both parents are

Figure 2a   How recessive inheritance works

a recessive disease increase if the parents are blood relations. This 1 in 4 type of inheritance is called Mendelian after a nineteenth-century monk who deduced it from his work with peas. It is sometimes misinterpreted to imply that if one child is born with a disease inherited in this way, a couple may then have three further children who will be unaffected. But the laws of heredity don't work like this. The 1 in 4 type of inheritance means that, for a couple each of whom are carriers of a recessive disease, each baby they have will have the same 1 in 4 chance of being affected. It can and does happen that 3 out of 3 children in the same family will have the same disease. Other examples of autosomal recessive disorders are sickle-

How Dominant inheritance works

One affected parent has a single faulty gene (**D**) which *dominates* its normal counterpart (**n**).

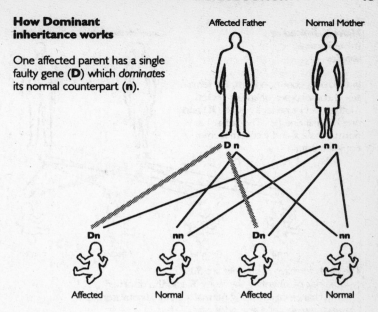

Each childs chances of inheriting either the **D** or the **n** from the affected parent are 50%

Figure 2b   How dominant inheritance works

cell disease, thalassaemia, Tay-Sachs disease and Friedrich's ataxia.

In another form of inheritance the abnormal gene will always override or dominate its normal counterpart. An example of an autosomal dominant disease inherited in this way is Huntington's chorea. There are about 2,000 diseases known to involve dominant inheritance. They affect both males and females and can often be traced through many generations of a family. The disorder is not transmitted by people who are unaffected themselves, but this apparently simple statement is confused by the fact that the effects of some dominant diseases are not seen until relatively late in life.

How X-linked inheritance works

In the most common form, the female sex chromosomes of an unaffected mother carry one faulty gene (**X**) and one normal one (**x**). The father has normal male x and y chromosome complement.

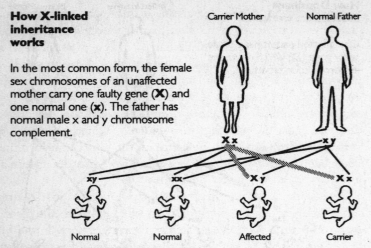

The odds for each *male* child are 50/50:
1. 50% risk of inheriting the faulty **X** and the disorder
2. 50% chance of inheriting normal x and y chromosomes
For each *female* child, the odds are:
1. 50% risk of inheriting one faulty **X**, to be a carrier like mother
2. 50% chance of inheriting no faulty gene

Figure 2c   How X-linked inheritance works

Affected individuals usually carry a normal gene as well as its disease-dictating partner and are said to be heterozygous for a particular condition. Homozygosity – where an individual has two copies of the abnormal gene – is rare. It can only happen if inherited from two individuals with the same disorder, which is in itself unusual, and in any case having two copies of the abnormal gene may be lethal. For instance, if two individuals with the form of dwarfism known as achondroplasia marry and have children, 1 in 4 of the children will be homozygous and die, 2 out of 4 will be heterozygous and affected, and 1 out of 4 unaffected. Thus 2 out of 3 living children will be affected.

There can be a wide spectrum of disability with dominant diseases, from people who seem hardly affected to people who are severely affected. Unfortunately it's not possible to say definitively from antenatal gene studies how severely an individual will be affected, simply whether they have the gene or not. As we explore in ensuing chapters, there are very significant ethical problems associated with the detection of diseases such as Huntington's chorea, which are fatal, but which don't occur until well into adult life. Other dominant disorders include adult polycystic kidney disorder, Noonan's syndrome and myotonic dystrophy.

Finally there is something called sex-linked or just X-linked inheritance in which only males are affected, with the disorder being transmitted through healthy female carriers. In the most common form the female sex chromosomes of an apparently unaffected mother carry one faulty gene and one normal gene. The faulty gene will be protected from being expressed by the other sex chromosome pair. However, when the other chromosome is a male Y, which is little and provides no pairing partner, the abnormal gene will be expressed. The most famous sex-linked disease is probably haemophilia. The family tree of Queen Victoria who was a carrier of this disease is shown here. Because the European royal families of the day intermarried so much, the disease spread quickly. The son of the last Tsar was a haemophiliac.

I have said that haemophilia spread quickly because of intermarriage. Consanguinity – that is, a relationship by blood – has considerable implications as far as genetic disease is concerned because everybody probably carries at least one harmful autosomal recessive gene. In marriage between first cousins, the chance of a baby inheriting from both parents the same harmful recessive gene that originated from one of the common grandparents and was transmitted down both sides of the family is 1 in 64. The babies born of incestuous relationships between first-degree relatives (e.g. brother and

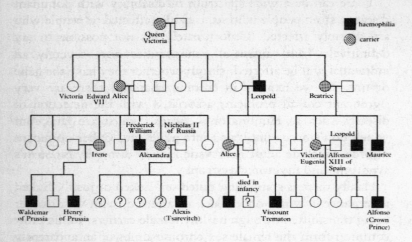

Figure 3 Family tree showing the transmission of the haemophilia gene in the Royal family. It probably arose as a mutation in Queen Victoria or her immediate ancestors, since she bore one afflicted son and two carrier daughters and there was no record of haemophilia in her ancestry. Males are represented by squares, females by circles in the chart. (*From* Biology A Functional Approach *Third Edition M.B.V. Roberts, Thomas Nelson & Sons Ltd 1982*

sister, father and daughter) are at high risk of severe abnormality. Only about half of the children born to first-degree relatives are normal.

Not all handicap in babies has the clear-cut inheritance that we have described, partly because it is the exception rather than the rule to have one characteristic controlled by one gene. Very often many genes work together, such as those responsible for skin colour. Sometimes you can have a gene, or more usually several genes working together, which would cause a particular problem if, and only if, the right environmental stimulus is present at the times when the genes are working.

This type of complex inheritance is called multifactorial inheritance and examples of problems caused include neural tube defects such as spina bifida, cleft palate and some congenital heart defects. You will of course immediately say, what environmental stimuli? Unfortunately nobody yet knows. But a more familiar example of genes being influenced by environment is that of height. A child with a gene that confers short stature is never going to be tall, but a child who might be tall may end up being only of average height because of factors such as illness or poor diet during his or her growth period. This is called the genetic potential, and it goes some way to explaining why, with better nutrition, children are taller today than they were 50 years ago.

Occasionally, faulty genes are not the result of inheritance but the result of mutations, that is faulty bits of the chemical code that arise spontaneously. These occur randomly. This is why screening of mothers at risk and abortion of babies affected by a particular genetic condition will never result in complete eradication of the condition. Achondroplasia (dwarfism) is a fairly frequent new mutation.

How do doctors go about finding one of these faulty genes? Sometimes geneticists know which chromosome the faulty gene appears on. They may also know the exact sequence of codons that make up the gene. If this is the case, the DNA can be extracted from a cell sample, and a specially engineered DNA probe introduced. You can think of a DNA probe as being rather like a sniffer dog. It will look for only one thing, a sequence of chemicals just like its own – perhaps the abnormal gene itself or perhaps a distinctive sequence of genes which are known to be close to an abnormal gene site. There are a number of DNA probes available for specific genetic diseases. Other methods of DNA analysis exist, dependent on the exact nature of the genetic defect being sought. I am deliberately omitting a more detailed discussion of DNA analysis because it is perhaps the fastest moving field of science

at present. What is written now will be out of date by the time
the manuscript is submitted, and woefully inadequate by
publication. Detailed information on the specific type of DNA
analysis is best obtained from genetic counsellors. You'll find a
list of all the regional genetic services at the back of this book.

Chromosomal Disorders

Before I finish the subject of genes, a further word is needed
about chromosomes which after all are the carriers of genes.
In all this talk about genes being passed down, and chromosome pairs in which one is inherited from the father and one
from the mother, you may end up thinking, well, why aren't
all daughters just like their mothers and all sons just like their
fathers? And our discussion to date has not indicated how
chromosome disorders can arise.

As we have seen, human cells contain 46 chromosomes,
organized into 22 so-called autosomal pairs, plus the sex
chromosomes, making 23 pairs in all. This is called the diploid
condition (regrettably genetics is full of such terms and they
are bandied about by doctors as if everyone knew exactly what
they were talking about, which is why I am introducing and
explaining them now). However, in sperm and egg, instead
of there being 23 pairs, there are 23 single chromosomes – the
so-called haploid number. This is a neat trick by the body as it
ensures that when sperm and egg meet, there are once again
the correct number of 23 pairs of chromosomes in the fertilized
egg. Sperm and eggs go through a special type of reducing
cell division called meiosis and this is when the infinite
variability that is the human condition occurs. Effectively the
deck is reshuffled. During meiosis, a cell splits into two (the
first meiotic division) and the two cells split again, resulting in
four new cells. Before the first split occurs, the DNA of each
chromosome replicates itself, so instead of there being a pair

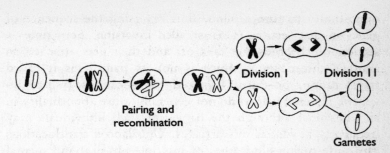

Figure 4 Meiosis (*From* ABC of Clinical Genetics *Helen M. Kingston, British Medical Journal 1990*)

of single chromosomes, there are a pair of doubles (called chromatids).

It is during the pairing up of the doubles that exchanges of information take place between one double member of a chromosome pair and its other half, ensuring a random shuffling of genes. During the intertwining of chromosomes, there is plenty of opportunity for all sorts of structural problems to arise. For example, a chromosome may break in two pieces and a section drop out, taking all its genes with it. The two ends then join up giving a chromosome which is shorter, but which has a bit missing. This is called a deletion. Most are lethal to the baby and will result in miscarriage but one where only a small piece of genetic material is lost causes the syndrome called Cri du Chat (from the noise made by the baby) in which the child is severely mentally and physically retarded. A variation on the deletion theme is where the chromosome forms itself into a ring, dropping a small portion as it does so. This 'ring' chromosome is responsible for one type of mental retardation syndrome.

Another kind of chromosome abnormality is where, when a chromosome breaks in two places, the middle section has an opportunity to turn around, thus reversing the sequence of genes in that section. This is called inversion. Sometimes a section of chromosome falls off and then gets attached to another chromosome which is not its pair. This is called translocation. So-called balanced translocations (where no genetic material is lost) do not generally cause abnormality in an individual although the babies of such individuals may frequently be lost as miscarriages. Unbalanced translocations can cause major syndromes of multiple physical and mental handicap. A variation on the translocation theme is called a Robertsonian translocation in which the breakpoints cannot be identified, but in which there are end-to-end fusions of chromosomes.

All these are structural problems that arise in sperm or egg. A further group of chromosome disorders are caused by a phenomenon called non-disjunction. What happens is this: instead of an orderly one chromosome of each pair going to each of a pair of new cells, one cell gets nothing, while the other gets an unseparated pair. Remember that this is going on as mature egg and sperm are being formed. The significance of this is that when sperm meets egg, and one of them already has a complete pair of one chromosome set due to non-disjunction, the addition of another chromosome is going to result in a threesome or trisomy. Down's syndrome is the best known trisomy but there are others – Edward's syndrome involves a trisomy of Chromosome 18, while Patau syndrome is a trisomy of Chromosome 13. A condition in which there is an odd number of chromosomes, either one less or one more than expected, is called aneuploidy.

Occasionally it is possible for an individual to have two different karyotypes, called mosaicism. This goes against everything that we have just been saying about every cell having exactly the same genetic information. However, it does sometimes happen because of non-disjunction during cell divisions in the developing embryo. The most usual form of

The total number of chromosomes is given first followed by the sex chromosomes

46 XX   normal female
46 XY   normal male
47 XXY   male with Klinefelter's syndrome
47 XXX   female with triple X syndrome

Additional chromosomes are indicated by a plus or minus

47 XY + 21   Male with trisomy 21 (i.e. Down's Syndrome)
46 XX + 12p   Female, additional matter on short arm of Chrom 21

Structural arrangements are described identifying the p & q arms and the location of the abnormality

46 XY del 11 (p13)   Deletion in short arm of Chrom 11 at band 13

Figure 5   Reporting of karyotypes

mosaicism is for Down's syndrome where some cells will have 46 chromosomes and others 47. The proportion of each type of cell line differs among different tissues of the body but also determines the phenotype. Thus, for Down's syndrome mosaicism, the characteristic facial appearance may not be present, although intelligence may be limited – or vice versa.

1   Routine Tests

Before going on to consider some of the specialized tests
available to women in pregnancy, it is worth explaining the
purpose of some of the other routine 'tests' which are undertaken during the course of your care. A recent review of
routine procedures during pregnancy revealed that many
mothers were not aware of their purpose; a significant proportion claimed to have had tests such as AFP (the screening test
for neural tube defects such as spina bifida) when in fact they
had not had them. It is difficult to be persistent about the
purpose of tests when you are lying like a beached whale,
partially dressed, but don't ever be afraid to ask, or be put off
by someone saying, 'It's just routine'. And it isn't always the
case that hospital staff are being patronizing when they say
something like this – they've probably seen how anxious a
woman can get if she is told that, for instance, her blood is
being tested for syphilis. The woman may immediately jump
to the conclusion that staff must think that she is at risk in
some way. On the contrary, syphilis testing is just what the
staff say it is – routine.

Here are the most usual types of routine testing undertaken
in pregnancy. If test results are not normal, further tests, either
repeats of the same test or variations on the same, may be
required to find why your test result wasn't as it should be.

TESTING YOUR URINE

You will be asked to give a urine sample for testing every time
you have an antenatal check-up. You will see this written in
your notes as an 'MSU', which stands for mid-stream urine.

The area around the vulva contains lots of contaminating organisms which will be swished into your sample if you give the nurse the very first bit of urine that you pass, whereas a mid-stream specimen will be a much more accurate reflection of the real contents of your urine. Giving a mid-stream specimen is something of an art as very few women know how long their stream of urine is likely to last, and by implication, the moment when they ought to start collecting their mid-stream specimen. Wait too long and you may run out of pee altogether. The trick is to drink a reasonable amount on the day of your check-up and then not pee until you arrive, making your MSU sample your first task.

The sample will be tested there and then for the presence of sugar and for protein, using special proprietary sticks which turn different colours depending on the amount of these substances present. Your first visit sample will also be cultured, usually just overnight, to see whether any bacteria are present. Subsequent visit specimens are not usually cultured unless there is a specific reason to do so, for instance, if you complain of a burning sensation when passing urine (dysuria) which might be indicative of infection. If this is the case, your urine will usually be cultured for a longer period of time than just overnight.

If the results are all normal, i.e. no sugar, no protein and no significant bacterial growth, 'NAD' will be written in your notes. This stands for 'no abnormality detected'.

Tests for sugars in urine

The way in which your body deals with sugars alters during pregnancy. Normally your body manages to keep your blood sugar levels within a fairly narrow range, no matter how many Mars Bar Ice Creams you have scoffed in an evening. Achieving this feat involves a series of body chemicals, one of the most important of which is the hormone insulin which has to be secreted in greater quantities than normal during pregnancy because of the anti-insulin effects of some of the pregnancy hormones. If insulin is not as effective in pregnancy, not all sugars are dealt with and may end up being dumped with the urine. Excretion of sugar in urine during pregnancy is common. This is the factual basis of several old wives' tales about how to tell if someone is pregnant, for instance, that if a spot of a woman's urine dries to leave a white mark (i.e. crystals of sugar) then she is likely to be pregnant. In some women, glucose tolerance will be impaired to such an extent that they become temporarily diabetic while they are pregnant (so-called gestational diabetes). In a very few women, pregnancy will reveal previously unrecognized diabetes.

You should be aware that sometimes, if you give a urine sample shortly after a heavy meal, sugars will be detected in your urine. There is nothing wrong – you just overloaded your system. But just to be sure, the usual practice in this instance is to repeat the test, on a further sample of urine, several hours later during which time you have eaten nothing further. If the second sample still shows the presence of sugar, it might be that your body isn't dealing with sugar in your system in the way that it should. To establish the true picture you will be asked to come back for a glucose tolerance test (GTT). A blood sample will be taken. You will then be given a measured amount of glucose to drink (often in the form of lukewarm Lucozade in a plastic cup). You will be asked to wait for a set amount of time (usually two hours) before a second blood sample is taken. The amounts of glucose contained in your blood before and after your glucose drink are then compared. A plasma glucose reading of less than 8 mmol per litre following a known glucose load is normal, between 8 and 11 indicates impaired glucose tolerance, while a reading greater than 11 would be indicative of diabetes. In some hospitals, a glucose tolerance test at the booking visit is

routine, while in others it may be offered routinely to those
with a first-degree relative with diabetes, those who are very
overweight and those who have had a previous baby who
weighed 10 lbs (4.5 kg) or more. Of course, none of these risk
factors means that you will develop diabetes in pregnancy, but
it is still worth checking.

Why does sugar matter so much? It is known that in poorly
controlled diabetics there is a greater miscarriage and perinatal
mortality rate. Babies of diabetics tend to be big (sometimes
in excess of 10 lbs or more) which may cause problems at the
time of delivery. Fetal lung maturation may be delayed giving
rise to breathing problems not dissimilar to those of very tiny
babies at birth. In women whose diabetes was under very
poor control in very early pregnancy, there is a greater chance
of fetal handicap. Having said all of this, it is important to
emphasize that there is no increase in congenital abnormalities
in women who develop abnormal glucose tolerance during
pregnancy. Meticulous control of blood sugar is the key to
minimizing fetal and maternal risks which is why the levels of
glucose in your urine are monitored so carefully by frequent
testing.

Protein

The presence of protein in the urine is measured with a
dipstick. It is rather a rough and ready sort of screening test,
but it is nevertheless vital in the prevention of a problem
specific to pregnancy, called eclampsia. This used to be called
toxaemia of pregnancy and you may also hear it called other
names such as pregnancy-induced hypertension. Eclampsia is
characterized by fits and is one of the most dangerous medical
emergencies in pregnancy. The phase that precedes eclampsia
is called pre-eclampsia. It is characterized by a range of
symptoms of which raised blood pressure, the appearance of
protein in the urine and oedema (a build-up of fluid) are the

most familiar. In the 1920s and 1930s, literally thousands of British women each year died as a result of eclampsia and even today it is still the largest single cause of maternal mortality. Eclampsia and pre-eclampsia cause the deaths of 1,000 babies a year in the UK and many thousands more babies are born smaller than they ought to be as a result of these syndromes. A detailed discussion of the causes of pre-eclampsia is outside the scope of this book, but should you want to know more, you should read an excellent paperback called *Pre-eclampsia, The Facts* (OUP, 1992) by Chris Redman and Isobel Walker.

The results of the proteinuria test are recorded as trace +, ++ and so on, up to 4 plusses. The test measures the concentration of protein in the urine, not the total amount, so if your urine is fairly concentrated (as it might be on a hot day), the number of plusses may be high but may not be as alarming as you might at first think. The 'trace' result is, in general, nothing to worry about at all. If your urine tests continued to indicate proteinuria, you may be taken into hospital for a 24-hour urine collection in which the total amount of protein being lost is measured. In general, you will feel perfectly well but you must take proteinuria seriously, especially if it is associated with high blood pressure. It is a clear sign that the function of your kidneys is beginning to deteriorate and that danger is imminent. Do not fight hospitalization in this situation. Accept that however well you feel, your body is sounding the clearest possible alarm bells on your behalf. The purpose of admission to hospital is not, however, as many people believe in these situations, for bed rest which actually has no value at all in terms of curing your problem. Pre-eclampsia is not a disease which runs a predictable course and while some women can have proteinuria and high blood pressure for some weeks without developing eclampsia, for others it merely provides a day or so of warning. The onset of eclampsia can be terrifyingly fast and the purpose of hospital admission is to ensure that you and your baby are monitored continuously. Only in this way can prompt action, such as early delivery, be taken, should it be necessary, to save the life of your baby and possibly yours too. (See also testing blood pressure.)

Bacteria

Testing for the presence of bacteria in urine is important for several reasons. Pregnant women are particularly liable to urinary tract infections. This is because women's urethras (the urethra is the tube that connects the bladder to the outside world) are very short – just 4 cm on average, compared to about 18 cm in men. During pregnancy, the vulval area is much moister than normal and provides an ideal breeding ground for bacteria which often ascend the urethra and colonize the bladder too. In addition, the rate of flow of urine is reduced in pregnancy, partly because your baby is sitting on your ureters (the tubes that lead from the kidneys to the bladder) and this also encourages bacterial growth. About 6 per cent of women attending antenatal clinics have infected urine, although they may have no other symptoms. Cystitis is a frequent complaint in pregnancy and any urinary tract infection needs prompt treatment as otherwise a nasty kidney infection called pyleonephritis may develop. Another reason for keeping a close watch on the bacterial count in the urine is that it has been postulated that some cases of premature labour may be the consequence of asymptomatic bacterial infection. For the same reason you may find that in your hospital vaginal swabs are taken at specific stages of pregnancy and antibiotic treatment offered if the count of one of several types of bacteria is high, even though you are perfectly well and have no symptoms of infection.

TESTING BLOOD PRESSURE

For the reasons we have outlined earlier relating to the detection of pre-eclampsia, regular blood pressure monitoring is essential in pregnancy. Contrary to popular belief, blood pressure actually falls during the early part of pregnancy. A normal blood pressure is about 110/70. The top reading is called the systolic pressure, and the bottom one, the diastolic pressure. Hospital admission is usually indicated if the diastolic reading is 100 or more – 140/90 is usually arbitrarily decided as the dividing line, although blood pressures greater than this may be tolerated if there are no other symptoms. Conversely, a blood pressure lower than this, if accompanied by several plusses of proteinuria, can be a cause for as much concern. It is true that more attention is paid to the diastolic figure (the bottom one) than to the upper, systolic figure which can fluctuate considerably with emotion, stress, etc.

Because we know high blood pressure is also called hypertension, there is a feeling that somehow it is caused by tension or nervousness. While blood pressure does fall during sleep and while, yes, it may rise temporarily in response to stress (such as a man in a white coat walking towards you to measure your blood pressure), the sustained high blood pressure that is characteristic of pre-eclampsia is nothing to do with stress. It is not brought on by 'overdoing things', by hard work, or by life crises such as moving house (something we all seem to want to attempt when pregnant). Ill-informed medical staff often suggest, when faced with a pregnant woman with high blood pressure, that she should 'take things easier', thereby implying that she has been the cause of her own problem. This is quite wrong. Chris Redman, Director of the Harris Birthright Centre for Pre-eclampsia in Oxford, suggests that you think of high blood pressure in pregnancy rather as you think of having a temperature. Relaxing may make you feel a bit better but until you cure the cause, your temperature will persist. Basically you are stuck with high blood pressure as long as you have a baby, and more importantly, a placenta, inside you. Having your blood pressure checked is probably the single most important test in pregnancy. It saves more lives than all other pregnancy tests put together, for there are no other visible symptoms of pre-eclampsia. Perhaps astonishingly for such a potentially serious condition, you will go on feeling perfectly well until the moment when it may be too late to do anything at all to save your baby. Never skip having your blood pressure tested.

Blood pressure by its very nature is not constant – it shoots up and down and rather perversely, when you think it should be lowest (for instance, when relaxing), it may be at its highest. If you have been lying down for some time before the reading is taken, a lower blood pressure may be recorded. This is because when you lie flat, the womb presses down on the blood vessel that returns blood to the heart, causing a temporary drop in blood pressure – so-called supine hypotension – which is why you may feel faint if you get up too quickly when you are heavily pregnant. The point to be made is that you should not be overly alarmed by the results of just one blood pressure reading. At least two or more readings should be taken, a little space apart in order to get a better picture of your blood pressure.

BLOOD TESTS

When you arrive for your first appointment at hospital, the so-called booking visit, blood will be taken. Hospitals vary in the 'routine' tests that they undertake on the initial blood sample but the following discussion indicates the most common ones. Obviously some, such as ABO blood groupings, are one-off but the results of others, like your rhesus grouping, may indicate the need for further blood testing throughout your pregnancy. Another set of routine blood testing is undertaken at about 28 weeks.

ABO Grouping and Rhesus Status

Your blood group will be checked (even though you may already know it). This is in case you need an emergency transfusion – if you are having a haemorrhage, there isn't time to hang about while somebody types your blood. A note is also made of your rhesus grouping, which is another type of blood group – either positive or negative. Most people in Britain (80 per cent) are rhesus positive. A problem can arise in pregnancy if the mother is rhesus negative and the baby is rhesus positive. The blood of the baby contains something called a D antigen, although the mother's does not. If the baby's blood gets into the mother's circulation (as it usually does at birth), the mother forms antibodies against the D antigen. These antibodies may affect future pregnancies by attacking the red blood cells of rhesus positive babies. However, these days, an anti-D injection is given within 72 hours of delivery which destroys any of the baby's blood cells that have entered the mother's circulation before they have had a chance to sensitize her. About 2 per cent of rhesus negative women will not be protected by anti-D following birth, since they will have already become sensitized following the leakage of a few fetal blood cells across the placenta. For this reason some centres give anti-D to rhesus negative women at 28 and 34 weeks. In any case, if you are rhesus negative, expect to have further blood tests during pregnancy to monitor your antibody status.

Testing for rhesus grouping is perhaps the perfect example of the benefit that routine testing of all women can bring. Forty years ago a rhesus negative mother might, with luck, have had one unaffected pregnancy. But all subsequent pregnancies would have been problematic, with the baby often being born with severe anaemia or even dying in utero. Today such problems are very rare indeed thanks to monitoring of the rhesus antibody. In the UK alone, perinatal mortality from rhesus haemolytic disease has fallen from about 560 a year in 1950 to about 23 per year today.

Blood count

Your haemoglobin level will be measured (haemoglobin is the red oxygen-carrying pigment of the blood) in case you either are anaemic, or as a baseline measurement should you later develop anaemia. Curiously those women who think they might be anaemic are often found to have quite normal haemoglobin levels, while quite serious degrees of anaemia may be tolerated by other women who assume that the general lassitude they experience is all to do with pregnancy. In general, iron supplements are not given routinely to all women these days as they are simply not necessary – most of the iron ending up quite literally going down the pan, but you will be offered iron if you are anaemic. Further blood investigations may be indicated if you are from an ethnic grouping in which haemoglobinopathies such as thalassaemia or sickle-cell anae-mia are common.

Rubella Antibody Status

All women are screened for the presence of rubella antibodies. Basically, if you have rubella antibodies you are immune and have no need to worry if you are in contact with rubella (German measles) cases during your pregnancy. If you are not immune, you should avoid contact with those with rubella and should ensure that you are immunized following the birth of your baby.

Toxoplasma Antibody Test

This is not a routine test because of the very large number of false positive results that it would generate were the current methods of testing to be used on a routine basis. Read Chapter 5 on toxoplasmosis for further information.

Wasserman Test

Unknown to most pregnant women, blood is routinely tested on booking for syphilis, the so-called Wasserman test. If syphilis in pregnancy is left untreated the baby may be born with congenital syphilis which causes mental retardation and bone abnormalities among other things.

HIV and Hepatitis Status

Many hospitals now test, on an anonymous basis, for antibodies to HIV. Non-anonymized testing may be offered to those with specific risk factors (bisexual or drug-using partner, recent visit to certain countries where AIDS is prevalent, etc.).

Some hospitals routinely test for Hepatitis B Surface Antigen (HBsAG). If the mother is an unknowing carrier of this antigen, the baby has a 70–90 per cent risk of becoming a chronic HBV carrier. Treatment of the newborn baby of a positive mother with hepatitis B immunoglobulin (HBIG) and hepatitis B (HB) vaccine is very effective in preventing the development of the HBV chronic carrier state.

WEIGHT

Finally, a routine test that is still carried out, though some clinics disagree with its value. Excessive weight gain or, alternatively, failure to gain weight can both be indicators of potential trouble in pregnancy, which is why many clinics still do it. One word, however, about weight gain. Some pregnancy books seem to suggest that weight is put on in a gradual and sustained way during pregnancy. It isn't like this in real life. One day you will wake up to find that it looks as though somebody has crept in during the night with a football pump, so enormous has your bump become seemingly overnight. If you have put on loads of weight between one visit and the next, don't panic. Providing that this weight gain isn't repeated at every visit (and it won't be), you will be fine. You may be comforted to know that there is a good deal of evidence to show that light women eat more and put on more weight in pregnancy than heavier women. Your height will also be measured on your first visit as height has to be related to weight in order to work out whether a woman is over-weight or not.

FAMILY HISTORY TAKING

In addition to all the tests mentioned so far, your booking visit is the time when a detailed family history is taken. You will be asked about your health, particularly in relation to current chronic disease (e.g. diabetes, renal problems, epilepsy, asthma, etc.), although if you have problems like these, I hope you will already have discussed the impact they may have on your pregnancy with your GP or specialist consultant prior to pregnancy. You will be asked whether you smoke, how much alcohol you drink and about the health of your partner and immediate family. If your parents or your partner's parents are dead, you may be asked for their cause of death. A history of diabetes in the family may be especially important in relation to pregnancy. You will be asked if there are any inherited illnesses. On the good news side, you will be asked whether there are twins in the family. Non-identical twins are known to be quite strongly familial. You will be asked about your job and your partner's job. You will be asked where you live and may be surprised to be asked how many rooms there are and what social support you have. All of these things, although they may seem rather personal, can play an import-ant part in the outcome of pregnancy. For instance, it is known that prematurity is more common in single teenage girls who have no one in whom they can confide.

If this is your second or subsequent pregnancy, you will have an obstetric record and the management of this preg-nancy and the range of tests offered to you will of course be influenced by what happened to you and your baby in your previous pregnancy.

'ROUTINE' ANTENATAL SCREENING OR DIAGNOSIS FOR FETAL HANDICAP

Hospitals vary enormously in what they offer in terms of 'routine' antenatal screening and diagnostic tests for fetal abnormality. Some hospitals offer routine triple test screening (see page 138), others offer AFP screening (see page 132), some do not offer either. Some hospitals offer one routine ultrasound scan (see page 8) at 16–18 weeks and another at 32 weeks, others only offer one scan at 20 weeks. Some hospitals will make amniocentesis (see page 104) available to all women over 35 years old, others only to women over 37 years old. Such policies have much more to do with available finance than with reasoned medical practice. The background to all of these different policies is given in each of the appropriate specialist chapters.

PRE-PREGNANCY TESTING

Pre-conceptual care has become increasingly popular in recent years with many prospective parents actively preparing themselves for pregnancy. There is no doubt that good health plays an important part in the outcome of pregnancy but good health is in itself no guarantee that you will have a healthy baby.

There are a number of specialist agencies which offer testing, often of hair, for specific deficiencies of minerals such as zinc prior to pregnancy, claiming that if mineral deficiencies are rectified, then the risks of handicap, miscarriage, stillbirth, etc. will be minimized. You should be extremely suspicious of these agencies. For a start, as I have repeatedly said in this book, no one can guarantee the outcome of pregnancy. You should also realize that the link between deficiency states and fetal handicap is often tenuous in the extreme. Take the well-documented story of folic acid. A recent Medical Research Council (MRC) trial has demonstrated conclusively that giving folic acid prior to and during early pregnancy to women who have already had one child with a neural tube defect (such as spina bifida) reduces subsequent cases of neural tube defects in this group of women by 70 per cent. So doesn't this prove that inadequate folic acid is the cause of neural tube defects? And shouldn't folic acid be given to all women prior to pregnancy? Such quantum leaps cannot be made. For instance, the problem could be not that these women all had inadequate folate intake but that they all shared an inherited inability to metabolize the dietary folate that was available to them. Just because some is good doesn't mean that a lot is better for everyone, although this appears to be the conclusion of a recent government report which recommended an additional 400 μg of folic acid per day for women around conception and in the first three months of pregnancy. The FDA in America have advised that total consumption should not exceed 1 milligramme per day, except under care of a doctor. In the same way, research findings that stillborn babies have abnormally low levels of zinc or tin or other minerals cannot be directly related to an inadequate intake by the mother of that particular mineral, either before or during pregnancy. This is discussed in more depth in Chapter 3, 'The Risk Ladder'.

And if you have had a previous miscarriage and are impressed by the statistics that these organizations quote, saying that the miscarriage rate among their clients is either far lower than the average or nil, just think about it. A woman who has had one miscarriage has a 95 per cent chance of a successful pregnancy next time around – so nine out of ten women who come for tests and 'treatment' with vitamin or mineral supplements are going to have a full term pregnancy next time around anyway, supplements or not.

What other pre-pregnancy tests are available? We discuss testing for Toxoplasma prior to pregnancy in Chapter 5. For the moment, you should be aware that testing for Toxoplasma has a high false positive rate. This means that you may be reassured that you are immune when in fact you are not. By all means have testing prior to pregnancy, but do not stop using common sense measures, such as washing your vegetables, avoiding handling contaminated cat litter, etc. just because you think you are immune.

All women should be tested for rubella antibody status prior to pregnancy. Rubella is almost completely preventable but when maternal infection does occur in early pregnancy it is very likely to cause damage to the baby. Cataracts, malformations of the heart and deafness are the best known of the malformations caused by rubella. Regardless of immunization, 80 per cent of British women are already immune to rubella by adulthood, but since this is one source of potential worry that you can actively avoid, have a rubella antibody test – even if you know you have had rubella vaccination in the past.

Pregnancy and kidney problems are very often not happy bedfellows. But it is frequently quite difficult for consultants to be specific about the risks to your future kidney function that may result from pregnancy. Recently, scientists at Newcastle University have been investigating something called the Renal Haemodynamic Reserve (RHR) which can provide a much more accurate picture of the severity or otherwise of kidney problems. Obviously, this kind of testing needs to be carried out before pregnancy if you are one of those unfortunate individuals who need to weigh up the risks to your future health of becoming pregnant.

In the section on risks, I have outlined those chronic disease states that can affect pregnancy outcome, such as diabetes, heart disease, epilepsy, etc. While women with these problems regularly have healthy babies despite their pregnancy being unplanned, it is far better, for your own peace of mind, to talk to your specialist consultant in advance of becoming pregnant. This is especially important for diabetics as it has been shown that immaculate sugar control prior to, and soon after, conception is the most effective way to lessen risks to both mother and baby. If you have a chronic condition your consultant may feel it appropriate to run some tests to establish your exact state of health prior to pregnancy. In this way, a baseline set of measurements can be obtained which can be compared to any taken during pregnancy.

Remember, there are at least 5,000 single gene defects. You or your partner could be, in fact very probably are, carriers of a lethal genetic disease. However, it makes no sense to try to test for carrier status before pregnancy because you simply don't know what you are looking for. The exception to this is cystic fibrosis. CF is Britain's most commonly inherited disease, with approximately 1 in 20 adults being carriers. About 95 per cent of CF babies are born to parents with no family history of the disease because, as I have shown before, carriers are perfectly healthy individuals. Mass screening may well be introduced before the end of the century. All that is required is a sample of your cells and these can be obtained by using a special mouthwash. If you would like to do this, you should contact the Cystic Fibrosis Research Trust (see page 189) who will advise you about the test, where to get it and about pre-test counselling.

Finally, if you have a history of inherited disease in the family, now is the time to find out whether you are a carrier. We explain about blood tests, linkage studies and family pedigrees in Chapter 8, 'Genetic Counselling'. If you know that you are at risk, an unplanned pregnancy may send you and your carers into a panic. It is far better to plan your pregnancy, discuss with specialists what tests are available and appropriate to the particular genetic problem, and then, the minute you are pregnant, timetable the tests. In this way, you will have time to prepare yourself.

2   To Test
or not to Test

To be pregnant is to be on an emotional rollercoaster. What
we feel about ourselves and about the baby we are carrying
changes not just by the day, but sometimes by the minute. At
one moment, we are very aware of the baby inside us, at
another, the baby seems remote and almost unreal. We may
become forgetful, tearful, unreasonable, and may feel quite
unable to think things through with any degree of clarity.
Despite all of this, pregnancy is the time when we are forced
to make major decisions which have the power to affect not
only our own lives but the lives of our partner and family too.
Many women think that they have come to terms with the
issues involved in antenatal testing prior to pregnancy, only to
find that being pregnant changes their perspectives entirely.
Don't expect to be consistent in your feelings about whether
to test or not. One moment you may be sure, and then with
bewildering speed you will change your mind. It is all part of
being pregnant.

This book can't take your decisions about testing for you. It
cannot tell you what is right and what is wrong, whether to
test or not. There is no correct answer for any given situation,
only what is right for you and your baby, and in the end you
are the only person who can decide that. What this book can
do is give you as much information as possible about testing
and allow you to draw your own conclusions.

For those faced with passing on a fatal disability, choices
about testing in pregnancy may be easy, although such
decisions will inevitably still prove distressing. For others,
choice is a great deal harder. Testing forces us to think about
things that we would perhaps rather not think about, such as
'Could I cope if my child was different?' You may prefer not

to think in this way, feeling instead that you will confront this question if and when you come to it. Some people might condemn this attitude as being 'head in the sand', of being irresponsible about the implications that taking up testing will inevitably bring. I don't think women should feel guilty about feeling this way. When you are not sure of your own feelings about such major issues, from hour to hour let alone from day to day, perhaps concentrating on the practical is a valid way of coping. If you are one of life's optimists, hoping never to have to cross your particular bridge, fine, but please read the specialist chapters carefully so you understand just what is involved.

One of the most important points about testing is to understand what the tests are for, what they can tell you and, just as importantly, what they can't tell you. There is more detailed information about each of the tests in the specialist chapters but for the moment you need to understand that a specific test, while answering one question, may leave others unanswered. For instance, amniocentesis or CVS will provide samples of the baby's cells. By preparing a karyotype (a spread of the chromosomes in a cell), a cytologist can say, with confidence, whether your baby is a boy or a girl, whether there are a normal number of chromosomes (thus excluding Down's syndrome which involves an extra chromosome) and whether the chromosomes are the normal size and shape. What the karyotype cannot tell the cytologist is whether your baby has a heart abnormality, or whether your baby has a single gene defect such as cystic fibrosis. Thus it is entirely possible to have a 'normal' amniocentesis result but still have a baby who is born with a major handicap. You need to be clear about this in advance.

'TESTING MEANS TERMINATION'

There are a number of myths about testing in pregnancy. The first is that testing means termination. It doesn't. The purpose of testing is to provide you with information about your baby on which to base choices about his or her future care. In my opinion, testing should be offered even to those women or couples who are completely opposed to termination. Finding out that your baby is, for instance, a Down's baby, allows you and your family to come to terms with a baby who will be different. It allows you time to plan for some of his or her special needs. In addition, if this baby should have some particular problems (many Down's babies have heart abnormalities, for instance), then you can plan to give birth in a hospital which has the surgical skills and facilities which may be vital to your baby's care. Finding out that your baby has a cleft palate is another clear instance where information obtained as a result of testing (in this case, a scan) can be of vital importance and in which termination is a very unlikely option. These days, surgical treatment of cleft palate is extremely advanced and is usually carried out within days of birth. Knowing that you are going to have a baby with this problem means that you can arrange to meet other mums who have been through the same thing. They can take you through specific difficulties that you are likely to experience, as well as reassure you that all will eventually be well, despite the rather alarming appearance of your baby at first sight. Finally, there are certain conditions which, if detected by tests, are amenable to treatment in utero. A scan may reveal that your baby is developing hydrops (an excessive collection of fluid), perhaps because of rhesus incompatibility; a series of intrauterine transfusions may well save your baby's life.

I have concentrated above on the negative aspects of testing, of discovering that all is not as it should be. Remember that testing is about good news too and that for the vast majority of mothers testing will provide reassurance that all is well. Such reassurance, however, is bought at a price, for testing will inevitably involve you in anxiety, either during or immediately after invasive testing such as an amnio ('Will I have a miscarriage?') and, for all tests, while you wait for the results. Sometimes the experience of tests that you thought were just routine or regarded almost as being fun – for instance, your initial ultrasound scan – can turn into a full blown panic attack if there is the smallest hint of a suggestion that something might be wrong. Never forget what the purpose of a test is.

The myth that testing means termination is further promoted by some doctors who refuse to allow their patients to have amniocentesis or even have screening such as triple test, unless they have agreed that they will have a termination in the event of handicap being discovered. The Royal College of Physicians in their 1989 report 'Prenatal diagnosis and genetic screening' strongly condemn this practice but it is nevertheless still prevalent.

What is so silly about blanket policies like this is that the results of tests are not black and white. In reality, there are all shades of grey in which different types of handicap, depending on their degree, will have different implications. There isn't just one answer. For instance, an amniocentesis might reveal that your baby has a chromosome configuration consistent with Klinefelter's syndrome. Your baby, a boy, will be quite normal, both physically and mentally, although it is possible that he might have a small degree of learning difficulty. However, because of the extra X chromosome, he will also be infertile. Would the obstetrician who insisted that you agree to termination if an abnormality was found, insist that you go through with it in the light of this finding?

Another reason for abhorring this policy of offering testing only to those who will agree in advance to termination is that it means that both you and your partner mentally cut yourselves off from your baby, refusing to become emotionally involved until you have a 'normal' test result in your hand. You may also delay telling parents and close friends about the pregnancy until you are over this 'hurdle'.

If your doctor or consultant is persistent in this attitude, by all means go along with it if that is what it takes to get testing, but please be reassured that no one can force you to have a termination. In fact, you are free to change your mind at any time, about termination and about whether to test or not. But you should never be made to feel guilty just because you want the information about your baby that testing can bring. There should be no preconditions – but sometimes, in reality, there are.

THINKING THAT YOU KNOW THE ANSWER

You may have come to pregnancy secure in your beliefs about testing. But as we have shown, once you are pregnant black and white can quickly change to grey. For instance, most of us have fairly clear feelings about termination for reasons of fetal sex alone. But listen to this woman's story. She is Nigerian, married to a Nigerian and they have lived in Britain for the last ten years.

'Ours wasn't an arranged marriage. We met in England and just really fell for each other. We got married and then we had two girls in fairly quick succession. Kojo loves the girls but I know that he wanted a boy. At first it wasn't really an issue, but then his family started to get involved, and began to pressure him about having a son. I got pregnant again but had a miscarriage. I remember asking the nurse whether it was a girl or boy and when she said a girl, I was glad. In Nigeria it is acceptable for men to take more than one wife and Kojo's family began to urge him to return to Nigeria and take another wife, to make sure that he had a boy. At first he resisted this but since my miscarriage, I haven't managed to conceive and I can see that, although he loves me and the girls, he is thinking about it seriously. I'd do anything to have a boy and stop him taking another wife, even if it meant having an abortion if I found out I was carrying a girl.'

How would you react if your partner said he would take another wife? As I have said, all shades of grey.

INVOLVING YOUR PARTNER

You need to involve your partner from the outset in your feelings about testing. Sometimes partners can be a wonderful source of support, sometimes, distressingly (because you always think they ought to be on your side), they take an opposing view. 'Don't expect me to stay around if you have a handicapped kid' was the parting shot of one father-to-be whose pregnant girlfriend felt ambivalent about testing. Unfortunately such attitudes are not uncommon. What people feel may be coloured by their own personal experience.

'I was 39 when I first became pregnant and wanted to have an amniocentesis. My husband agreed but he felt immensely guilty about this decision because his brother had Down's syndrome and he loved him dearly. For him, me wanting to have testing meant wiping out what he felt about his brother. I did have testing and the baby didn't have Down's but it was a very difficult time between us both, when it should have been wonderful.'

One of the most supportive things that a partner can do is to help you reason through what you feel about testing. If he takes the opposite viewpoint to yours and then perhaps you swap roles in the argument, you may end up with a clearer picture. On the other hand, you may both end up feeling more confused than ever but at least he will understand better how you feel. Mothers and mothers-in-law may completely fail in the understanding stakes, partly because antenatal testing is so foreign to them. In the main, anyone reading this book who is pregnant will not have a mother who experienced testing during her pregnancy. Very often the attitude is one of 'Well, I managed to have four perfectly healthy babies without all this fuss.' It may be true – but luck and statistics were on her side.

TESTING – THE DOMINO EFFECT

Deciding whether or not to have screening tests such as MSAFP (see page 132) may seem relatively easy. After all, the test is non-invasive, carries no risk to you or the baby and everyone else seems to be having it too. However, you should be aware that such tests can have a domino effect, where the discovery of a positive result – in this case, a raised AFP level – can lead to much more invasive forms of testing, such as amniocentesis, which you may previously have decided to reject. Once you have been given the information which by agreeing to the screening test you in effect requested there is no turning back. Of course you could just decide to go no further but in practice this means spending the rest of your pregnancy worrying about your baby now that such a potentially serious question mark has been raised. You may wish, as you go through a period in which you are acutely anxious, that you had never got involved with testing in the first place.

NOT HAVING TESTS – EMOTIONAL BLACKMAIL

We are all very much influenced by our own personal experience of handicap. If you have no handicap in your family, if all of your close friends have had normal babies, you may feel that handicap is a remote possibility. You may feel that since most babies are born healthy, there is no reason why yours shouldn't be healthy too. And of course, you would be right, because 39 out of every 40 babies born in Britain are indeed quite normal. You may feel that testing involves too much pressure and anxiety and that you would rather find out about your baby when he or she is born. If this is your view, then you should be supported in it. However, you may find that you are subject to all sorts of emotional blackmail from your friends and family. Worst, and most hurtful of all, is when the pressure comes from your partner. Thoughtless remarks such as 'What would you feel like if your baby was born with a handicap?' are made and suddenly the decision that you took to avoid stress and pressure is causing just that, stress and pressure. Probably the best thing to do in this situation is to find someone else who shares your views. There is nothing so lonely as being on your own in pregnancy. If you don't know anyone who feels as you do, organizations such as LIFE or the Society for the Protection of the Unborn Child (their details are at the back of this book) will listen to and support you.

GETTING TESTS

Contrary to popular belief, no mother can insist on testing the pregnancy. You may feel very strongly about wanting to have tests but in the end, particularly if the procedure is an invasive one such as amnio or CVS with a significant risk of miscarriage, doctors can refuse. Of course, you can circumvent the health service and go privately (amnios cost about £250) but you should be aware of the risk to your baby. Sometimes doctors recognize that for family reasons a woman may be particularly agitated or distressed about the possibility of an abnormal baby and then, even though the woman may be far younger than those who would normally be included in the amniocentesis programme, will arrange for amniocentesis. If you feel very strongly, try to arrange a time when you can talk to the consultant about your fears and concerns. He or she may prove to be more sympathetic than you had imagined.

Your hospital may or may not offer screening tests such as AFP or triple test. Again, you can arrange to have these privately but you should make sure, before you have these tests, that you know what to expect from the results and more importantly who to turn to if the result is abnormal.

THE PERFECT BABY

We all get consumed by an attack of what I call 'broderie anglaise fever' when we are pregnant. We have a rosy romantic view, which is entirely dispelled once you have had one child, of our smiling, sleeping, perfect baby in its gleaming, fresh crib with its broderie anglaise trim. We want our baby to fit into this rosy picture, to be perfect. In reality, of course, life isn't like this. None of us are perfect. Although we may dream in pregnancy that our babies will be brain surgeons or film stars or millionaires able to keep their doting mummies in a style to which they would like to become accustomed, in the end, our babies will be what they will be. Testing is often equated with the quest for the perfect baby – wrongly I believe, because in reality parents want the best for their baby, not for them to be perfect. These two things are not the same at all.

Having read all these dilemmas, now read the specialist chapters. Be sure before you commit yourself that you know what the test is for, what the implications are, what the test can reveal and what it can't. And remember, you can always say no at any stage.

3   The Risk Ladder

A medical journal recently carried a study about the risks of being hit by lightning. The authors of the paper had reviewed a large number of reported lightning strikes and concluded that those at minimal risk were individuals aged less than 6 or more than 90, who were non-smokers, who went outside only between September and May, avoiding trees, golf courses, football pitches and anywhere in Hertfordshire. Does this mean that if you are a 32-year-old smoker you should cancel your planned visit to the golf course in St Albans in July? Of course it doesn't. Unless you are sheltering from a storm, beneath the only tree for miles, the risk of being hit by lightning is not one that would normally disturb our sleep. We know that there is a theoretical risk of course, but life has to go on, thunderstorms or not, and we just have to go out and get on with it. In other words, although we are aware of the statistics of risk, we can be rational about them. But it is difficult, if not impossible, to be rational about risk in pregnancy. To be quoted a risk of 1 in 500 of one's baby being born with a handicap means nothing to us when we are pregnant. What we really want to know is what chance has my baby got of being that 1 baby in 500? For the record, every one of the 500 has the same risk of being *the* 1 in 500 – but the question still haunts us all the same.

One of the most difficult aspects of assessing risk, and therefore our needs for testing in pregnancy, is separating the wood from the trees. It is all too easy to get hung up about something which in the general scheme of things is of no importance, while ignoring something else which may be of far greater concern. I remember a lady calling me during a radio phone-in one day. She had heard of the dangers of taking drugs in pregnancy and was consumed with worry because she had taken two Strepsils when she was about eight weeks pregnant. She wanted information about antenatal diagnosis as she was convinced that her baby would have some major malformation. As she spoke, she began to sob. 'I can't think of anything else,' she said, 'except the fact that I might have been responsible for damaging my baby.' It then transpired that she was smoking 30 cigarettes a day to 'calm her nerves'. The Strepsils were of no importance at all, but her 30-a-day cigarette habit was a very real danger to her baby.

This story tells us just as much about pregnancy as it does about risk assessment. As far as potential risk is concerned, there is a conflict between wanting to know and not wanting to know. Wanting to know can become an obsession with a woman seeking information from a wide variety of sources only to discover that far from being the anxiety-reducing reassurance she sought it poses far more questions than it answers. For instance, it is thought that about 2 per cent of developmental defects are the result of exposure to drugs and other teratogens. While of initial comfort, the next question, 'And what about the rest?' brings the revelation that the cause of 70 per cent of congenital malformation is unknown. So how can we be sure about the 2 per cent? The answer is that we can't.

From the outset you must accept that sometimes there may not be an answer to your query about risk – or rather there is, but it is 'We don't know'. In the past, it was possible for doctors to make sweeping statements based on a relatively small amount of knowledge. Our understanding of the human body is now greater than ever before. And while such knowledge is a bright light, it also serves to throw into sharp relief areas about which we know very little. It is always said you have only begun to understand a subject when you realize that you know almost nothing in comparison to that which still remains to be understood. Nothing could be more true of pregnancy and the causes of handicapping conditions.

'We don't know' is an honest if ultimately unhelpful answer to a query about the risk of handicap. At the other end of the scale is the 'You'll be fine' type of response. There are of course lots of questions about risk which can be answered accurately but nevertheless this 'You'll be fine' airiness is, paradoxically, unsettling because you then begin to wonder whether this reassurance is based on solid science rather than just on goodwill. What we want in pregnancy are facts, figures and the latest studies. Pregnant women are the ultimate information consumers.

It has to be said that the quality of information that women receive in reply to enquiries about risk and whether they either should or needn't consider testing is not always all it ought to be. Frequently carers may not be up to date with the latest information. For instance, as you will read later, it has now been shown by numerous studies that there is no danger to the babies of pregnant women who use VDUs. Yet, for sure, despite statements from both the Health and Safety Executive and the Royal College of Obstetricians and Gynaecologists to this effect, some obstetricians and GPs will still be advising pregnant women to the contrary.

Remember, when you seek information about risk in pregnancy, GPs in particular are not and cannot be human encyclopaedias. Although they will each have their own area of expertise and experience, it may well not encompass your query, particularly if it is one that is a little off the beaten path. In medicine, it is often more important to know where to look for knowledge than to have the knowledge itself. And while your doctor may be aware of one particular well-publicized study that is relevant to your query, a specialist may know of several more studies and more importantly be able to provide an overview of their results (which are very often contradictory because of their differing study designs) in a far more effective way. In other words, asking your GP where to go for information, rather than expecting him or her to have it instantly to hand, may be a more effective route to real reassurance.

Women often say that their attitudes change once they have had a baby. Issues like global warming or the threat of nuclear war, which may have passed them by in the past, suddenly assume an urgent importance. The instinct to protect our young becomes paramount. The first waking of this instinct occurs in pregnancy, when risks which we would have dismissed just a few months ago begin to assume a major and very often unwarranted importance because of their possible effect on the baby inside us. Some of this worry is quite needless – but perhaps, as I have suggested, the urge to worry and to protect is sometimes one of instinct rather than rationality.

Each of us who has been pregnant will admit, usually well after the event, that in addition to what might be called legitimate worries, there were also other things which we knew were a bit silly, but which nevertheless assumed a major importance. Part of the problem with such worries is that while we are prepared to share some of our concerns with our GP or midwife, these others (which are just as real to us) are hugged to ourselves, as we fear the brisk 'Don't be so silly' response that our more logical selves reason that we might receive.

In my work as an agony aunt I get to hear many of these sort of all-consuming but usually quite groundless worries. Typical is one I hear frequently about Teflon: is ingesting flakes of Teflon from a past-its-sell-by-date non-stick frying pan harmful to the baby? For the record, no, it's not. Teflon is an inert substance, and eating a teaspoonful of Teflon is much akin to eating a spoonful of sand – it just passes straight through. All I can say to you about these concerns is get them off your chest if you possibly can.

One final point about risk. In a world without pollutants or nuclear weapons, in which every woman was adequately nourished and in which all those elements which we consider to constitute 'risk' were absent, there would still be women who had abnormal babies. Humans are no different from all other animals. There is no such thing as perfect reproductive efficiency – fetal wastage, be it as miscarriage or the death of the baby as a result of abnormality, is part of reproductive life's rich tapestry. We have forgotten that and have an unrealistic expectation that every pregnancy will go uneventfully to term, producing a perfect baby in the process. More than that, we believe that if this isn't the case then we must have done something wrong. While it makes sense to do what we can to avoid what is avoidable, there is a baseline which our best efforts will not be able to take us past. And although this baseline may represent our species' reproduction at its most efficient, it will still include pregnancies that end before they should and babies that are not perfect. Such is life.

The aim of this chapter is to review all those 'risks' that are associated with pregnancy, specifically those which might be responsible for causing damage to the baby, and to put them into some sort of perspective. You should be aware as you read that this information was put together at the beginning of 1993 and that while most of it will still be relevant, some information will have been superseded as a result of newly published research. If you have a specific query about pregnancy and want to be sure about getting the latest information, you should address your query to one of the specialist agencies listed at the end of this book. Armed with this information about risk, I hope you will be able to make more sense of your own needs as far as testing in pregnancy is concerned.

It has to be said that our assessment of what constitutes risk is very much affected by the amount of 'alarm input' we have received either consciously or subconsciously from the media and other sources. One example will suffice. Radiation workers receive on average about 1.4 milli-sieverts of radiation each year and have, on this basis, a risk of approximately 1 in 57,000 of developing cancer. In comparison, the risk of death from accident in the fishing industry is 1 in 800, and 1 in 6,000 for mining. If you are over 40, your risk of death from natural causes is 1 in 850 and if you smoke twenty cigarettes a day, you have a 1 in 200 chance of death. But ask ordinary people whether it is more dangerous to work with radiation or smoke ten cigarettes a day and I can guarantee that nine out of ten would give working with radiation as their answer. As I said, the assessment of risk is subjective.

If you have been deemed to be at 'high risk', it does not mean that you are going to have a handicapped baby, any more than being at 'low risk' guarantees that you will have a healthy baby. You have simply been put in a convenient medical pigeonhole, along with thousands if not hundreds of thousands of other women who are all deemed to be equal, because of their age or their race or their medical history. But we are not all the same, we are complex organisms, each of which is unique. We will not all react identically to the challenge that is pregnancy. Therefore estimates of risk can only be generalizations, based on our knowledge of how to deal with statistics, not copper-bottomed guarantees of the way that your baby will develop. Only when we have a 'history', after our first experience of pregnancy, can medicine attempt to be more accurate in its pigeonholing.

Our history may be the ultimate arbiter of risk, but nevertheless there are other risks which loom as large, if not larger, in the public consciousness and which you may be especially concerned about because of their prominence in the media. In reality, they may come fairly low down the risk ladder. Let us consider these first and then conclude with those things which may put women into the highest risk categories as far as possible abnormality in their baby is concerned. You may like to make a mental note – 'Yes, this applies to me', or 'This isn't me' – against each risk as you read through this chapter in order to come to some sort of self-assessment of risk.

NUTRITION PRIOR TO AND DURING PREGNANCY

The foreword to a recent book about planning a pregnancy by the pre-conceptual care group Foresight contained the statement, 'Our experience leads us to believe that most of the damage and ill-health that afflicts the unborn can be pre-empted if certain measures are taken in time.' The book went on to explain 'the vital importance of nutrition in pregnancy', citing inadequacies in various vitamins and minerals as being the cause of a whole range of fetal malformations. From this approach, which would almost seem to suggest that a pre-pregnancy and pregnancy unsupplemented by additional vitamins cannot result in a healthy baby, one can go to the other extreme where mother and developing baby are portrayed as a resilient unit in which the baby plays the part of parasite, taking all the nutrients it requires at the mother's expense, with handicap as a result of inadequate maternal diet a very rare event. Given that pregnant women may have heard both versions of this story, it is not surprising that nutrition, as far as most women are concerned, occupies a far higher rung on the risk ladder than it probably warrants, certainly as far as readers of this book are concerned.

There are three main areas of concern about nutrition prior to and during pregnancy: the avoidance of congenital abnormalities, having a diet which is sufficient to ensure that the baby grows properly and, finally, avoidance of infection with food-borne organisms such as Listeria, Salmonella and Toxoplasma.

Infection with Toxoplasma is discussed at greater length in Chapter 5. Infection with Listeria is not associated with fetal abnormality although listeriosis is a cause of premature labour, which may bring its own problems for the baby. Luckily listeriosis is a rare infection. Minimizing the risks of being infected by such organisms is in fact a personal creed for lifelong practice, not just something for use in pregnancy alone. Washing your hands after using the toilet (the Listeria organism, for instance, is often found in human faeces), washing your hands before eating, keeping pets away from surfaces used for food preparation, washing soil-grown vegetables before eating, adequately refrigerating perishable food and reheating cooked food thoroughly are all common sense measures which you should not only adopt yourself but also instil in your children for the sake of their future health.

The impact of pre-pregnancy weight and pregnancy weight gain on infant birth outcome, particularly on infant birthweight, is dramatic. Birthweight is not only a major determinant as far as a baby's immediate health prospects at birth are concerned, but also of its health prospects for life. Low birthweight is, according to recent work by Professor David Barker and the MRC Epidemiology Unit in Southampton, the principal risk factor in the development of coronary heart disease in later life. Providing that you are not very underweight because of an eating disorder or other problem (and remember that fertility is usually impaired in these situations, preventing pregnancy), it is highly unlikely, as an educated and motivated woman, that your baby is at risk of low birthweight because of poor nutritional status on your part. It would appear that nutritional status of the mother at conception is a more important determinant of a baby's birthweight than nutritional intake during the early months of pregnancy.

This fact may be of comfort to those of you who may actually lose weight in early pregnancy as you struggle to cope with the appetite loss and vomiting that morning sickness brings in its wake.

If, following an ultrasound scan, it is shown that your baby is perhaps smaller than it ought to be for the stage of pregnancy, you may thereafter have ultrasound scans on a weekly basis to monitor the baby's growth. However, as far as growth is concerned, remember that it is not just food intake that determines a baby's size. There are many reasons why babies may not grow properly in the womb – a well-known example is when the mother has the combination of high blood pressure and other factors known as pre-eclampsia (see Chapter 1). Sometimes there seems to be no obvious cause to explain poor growth in the baby and the mother may begin to worry that it must be because her diet is in some way deficient. Recent discoveries about the regulation of growth in babies may be helpful. Sometimes, instead of inheriting one of each chromosome pair from the father and one from the mother, both members of a pair of chromosomes are inherited from one parent. It appears that this phenomenon, known as uniparental disomy, may be a possible cause of hitherto unexplained poor fetal growth, especially if the chromosome pair are paternal, as inheritance of the mother's chromosome seems to be the more important determinant of growth regulation.

What of food, or lack of specific elements of food, being the cause of handicap? The risks of poor pregnancy outcome increase dramatically with decreasing social class. Because a woman is six times more likely to bear a handicapped baby if she is from the lowest as compared to the highest social class, and because poor diet is associated with poverty, it would seem logical to assume that poor diet plays a major part in handicapping conditions. Life, however, is not as simple. Women in the lowest social classes are more likely to smoke, to have higher intakes of alcohol, and have higher rates of infection due to poor hygiene and living conditions. All of these things, not to mention a multiplicity of social conditions such as lack of access to education or health facilities, are confounding variables which do not allow a simple relationship between diet and pregnancy outcome to be made. It is probably true to say that pregnancy outcome is rather like the pointer on one of those old-fashioned balance scales. Smoking may not be as important a risk factor if those things on the positive side of your health balance, such as good diet, lack of alcohol and good education, are heavily stacked. But poor diet added to an already groaning negative balance may tip the scales heavily in favour of a poor outcome.

Recently the results of the MRC trial on vitamin supplementation in the pre-pregnancy period have been published. The study related to women who had previously had a baby with a neural tube defect (NTD), such as spina bifida. Pre-pregnancy supplements of folate only and multi-vitamins and folate were shown to reduce the incidence of a subsequent affected pregnancy by over 70 per cent. Does this study not therefore show the necessity of good nutrition in general and of pre-pregnancy vitamin supplementation for all women in particular? Well, no, it doesn't. Neural tube defects are known to be multifactorial in origin, which means that while there is an inherited risk this may not necessarily be translated into an affected baby without the presence of another factor, such as an environmental agent (which is as yet unknown). Not all women who have a baby with an NTD have a diet lacking in folate. It may simply be that they have inherited a gene which does not allow them to use the folate in their diet as effectively as other women.

While on the subject of food and neural tube defects, there is no truth in the assertion that eating the green bits in potatoes causes this type of handicap. You should not eat the green bits of potatoes but only because the potato, like all the other members of its family which includes Deadly Nightshade, contains poisons (solanoids) in its green parts. The reason that potatoes got this reputation was because, as explained more fully elsewhere, neural tube defects occur more frequently in some parts of the UK than others. A common feature of all the high incidence areas, such as Northern Ireland and South Wales, was a diet which included large quantities of potatoes. It was an attempt to exploit this fact that led to the green potato scare, subsequently shown to be quite false.

Studying particular micronutrients such as folate or iron and whether supplements in pregnancy might prevent handicap is fraught with difficulties. Low maternal levels of zinc in particular have been cited as a cause of neural tube defects and numerous other congenital abnormalities, so it is worth taking you through the zinc story when trying to explain why supplements may not be the answer to 'deficiencies'. However, to start at the beginning, how do you define low zinc intake? In general, the dietary requirements for micronutrients in pregnancy are based on non-pregnant needs plus some – which was how a recommended daily allowance of 20 mg zinc came to be recommended. Dietary intake of zinc has been measured in many studies and in almost all of them it has been found to be much less than the recommended dietary allowance (in fact about 50 per cent of that recommended). The intake of micronutrients tends to parallel protein intake and zinc intake in particular is closely linked to that of protein. Thus, if diets were truly zinc deficient, it is also highly likely that there would be a parallel very low intake of protein. This is not the case. In order to take in as much zinc as possible, a protein intake of some 120 g (about 5 oz) would be required each day which would be a struggle for someone in the USA or the UK, and virtually unheard of in the developing world, where millions of women still have perfectly healthy babies.

Nevertheless, worry about zinc-deficient intakes is fuelled by the fact that the concentration of zinc in the mother's blood falls steadily as her pregnancy progresses, leading to 'zinc deficiency' by the time she delivers. In fact, measurement of zinc levels (and indeed of many other components of the mother's blood) is not a straightforward exercise because the blood becomes much more dilute in pregnancy. But if you measure zinc on a weight-for-weight basis, rather than just its concentration in blood, it actually stays the same throughout pregnancy and is not 'deficient' at all. On this evidence it would seem that zinc supplementation is unnecessary.

The effect of giving zinc supplements in pregnancy has in fact been studied and they do not prevent the fall in plasma zinc that occurs in pregnancy. It would appear that, partly because a pregnant woman's gut becomes much more absorbent, any additional zinc given is simply excreted. So zinc supplements have no effect – are they actually harmful? There is more and more evidence that micronutrients interact in the gut where an excess of one may lead to an alteration, perhaps a decrease in the absorption, of another. Iron, folic acid and alcohol have all been shown to affect adversely the intestinal absorption of zinc. Thus supplementation does not necessarily achieve the desired effect and may actually be counterproductive. It is much more appropriate that women who fall into a particular risk group, such as those who have had a previous pregnancy affected by an NTD, should be given extra vitamins.

One vitamin in particular, Vitamin A, is known to be extremely dangerous in excess in pregnancy and it is discussed later in the section on teratogens. Unless you are advised to do so for medical reasons, there is no need to take supplements prior to pregnancy.

Caffeine

Many women with an ongoing love affair with coffee find that one of the first signs of pregnancy is that they go right off it. It has been argued that this is an example of a biological protective mechanism and there has been some suggestion that a very high intake of coffee (more than 7 cups a day) is related to a decrease in infant birthweight. There is, however, no suggestion that caffeine is linked to human birth defects.

RADIATION

When we think of radiation, we think of Chernobyl, of hazardous emissions, of danger. In actual fact, radiation is all around us, and is both naturally and artificially produced. A whole spectrum of radiation exists, encompassing both electric and magnetic waves. The spectrum is based on the frequency and the wavelength of the radiation. Visible light is found in the middle of the spectrum. Although we see light as being white, it comes in a rainbow of colours which are exposed when white light is scattered, for instance when sunlight falls on raindrops. Near the violet end of this visible spectrum are found ultraviolet rays (responsible for tanning) and also X-rays and gamma rays. These latter rays are called ionizing radiation because of their ability to form charged particles as they break up material through which they are passing. At the other end of the spectrum are infra red, micro- and radio waves.

As far as pregnancy is concerned, ionizing radiation is of the greatest concern because of the very well documented ability of radiation to cause inherited defects in the offspring of exposed individuals – so let's tackle this one first.

We live on a radioactive planet. The earth itself is radioactive with further radiation reaching it from outer space. Thus everyone is exposed to natural radiation. In fact, we are exposed to 1,870 micro-sieverts a year from natural sources, compared to just 280 micro-sieverts a year from artificial sources such as X-rays. Weapons fall-out accounts for only 10 micro-sieverts annually. The scale of our exposure to natural radiation is awesome. For instance, the average person inhales over 30,000 radioactive atoms of radon, polonium, lead and bismuth per hour, which disintegrate giving off alpha and beta particles, as well as gamma rays. In the daily diet, some 7,000 atoms of uranium disintegrate every hour inside each of us. Natural radiation is all around us. We cannot escape it by going indoors and in some areas, notably those where homes are built of granite, the amounts of radiation indoors may be higher than outside because the materials used for building are themselves radioactive, or because the underlying substrate causes radioactive radon gas to enter the home. It is estimated that natural radiation is responsible for some 2,000 out of the 160,000 cancer deaths each year in the UK.

X-rays in pregnancy

Radiation does not affect all body tissues equally. Some are more sensitive than others, including the testes and ovaries where there is a known risk of serious genetic damage. The way in which radiation causes its damage to DNA is not yet fully understood, nor is the way in which DNA repairs itself on most occasions and does not progress to malignancy, mutation or alterations in the genetic code. While it is obvious that all ionizing radiation is harmful, it is also true that small amounts are less so. While the annual natural radiation intake is 1,870 micro-sieverts, the average chest X-ray gives a dose equivalent to about 20 micro-sieverts. This dose is lower than that given in the past when irradiation of the baby during pregnancy was associated with risks of childhood leukaemia. The 'ten day rule' whereby X-ray examination of the abdomen and pelvis in women of reproductive age is limited to the 10 days following a period has reduced the risk of inadvertent exposure to X-ray during pregnancy. However, it does sometimes happen and it will naturally be a cause for concern. The risk of damage is in fact very slight. It was recently concluded that there would be two extra cases of congenital handicap, usually mental retardation, for every baby exposed to 50 millisieverts (50,000 micro-sieverts) of radiation as an embryo – remember, a chest X-ray involves absorption of just 20 micro-sieverts.

The fall in risk from radiological exposure has largely been due to advances in equipment. Automatic exposure, improvements in X-ray film, etc. have meant that doses can be reduced. Most hospitals are equipped with modern machinery but some dental practices may have less up-to-date equipment, with a consequent higher level of radiation absorption. Dentists are not always as rigorous about the imposition of the ten day rule either. Even so, absorption from a dental X-ray remains minute in comparison with exposure to natural radiation. You absorb 10 micro-sieverts in cosmic radiation flying from Heathrow to Malaga airport. Let me herewith stake my claim to clairvoyance and say that a future pregnancy scare will involve the risk to women of reproductive age making frequent trips in planes, thereby increasing their exposure to cosmic radiation. Can I counter it in advance, however, by saying that no study (and people have looked) has shown an increased congenital handicap in babies born to air hostesses.

Video display units

In the early eighties, the first reports came in of adverse pregnancy outcomes in groups of women using video display units (VDUs). The cathode ray tube in a VDU emits radiation in the extremely low and very low frequency range. The possibility that close and continuous contact with this source of radiation was the cause of reproductive problems was extensively investigated and there were a very large number of studies. Initially the results were confusing. Although none of the studies showed an increase in handicap among babies born to women who had used VDUs extensively in pregnancy, some studies did seem to show an increase in the rate of spontaneous miscarriage. However, many of the studies were thought to be biased in that the VDU users were compared to groups of women who, although they worked in offices, were able to move around more and who were less stressed. In particular there were suspicions that the increased miscarriage rate might have been due to long hours in an uncomfortable sedentary posture, rather than to the VDUs. In 1991 the National Institute for Occupational Safety and Health completed a large and very careful study in the States which involved two groups of telephone operators, each with similar conditions and workstations, only one of which worked with VDUs. The study showed clearly that there was no difference in miscarriage rates. Another British study, which appeared in the British Journal of Industrial Medicine in 1992, reported similar results and concluded by saying that there was no justification for any further research in this area. Women who work with VDUs are not at increased risk of miscarriage and neither are they at extra risk of having babies with a handicap. Thus 12 years of uncertainty and worry about VDUs came to an end.

Televisions are a source of a very small amount of radiation but modern television screens are well shielded and you can be assured that they present no hazard.

Exposure to heat

There have been a number of scare stories recently about the risks to the baby of excessive heat (hyperthermia, another form of radiation) when a pregnant woman uses a sauna or takes a very hot bath. Specifically an increase in the number of neural tube defects such as spina bifida is mentioned. It is known that hyperthermia causes damage to the unborn baby in animal studies and that high body temperatures caused by fever can damage human babies, particularly in the first trimester (see infection, page 79). However, to compare this situation directly with hot baths etc. not only ignores some basic physiology but also, as my mother would say, assumes that we all stood behind the door when common sense was given out. First, the physiology. Our bodies are engaged in a constant round of activity in order to ensure that our core body temperature remains steady, no matter how hot or cold it is outside the body. Furthermore, during only moderate exercise the human body produces internally about 5 watts of energy per kilogram of bodyweight. This amount of energy would cause the body temperature to be raised by 1 degree in 12 minutes. The fact that we do not all die of heatstroke following a quick burst of hoovering is proof enough of our extraordinary capacity to control large temperature gains, be they produced inside or outside the body, by rapidly and efficiently organizing heat loss through blood cooling and other means. Even if a hot bath were sufficient to raise external skin temperatures by a degree or two, core body temperatures would not have changed one jot – and remember that your baby is safely ensconced in the body's core. And back to common sense – if high external temperatures were dangerous, how come millions of women who live in hot climates have healthy babies? And what's more, how is it that Finland, where taking saunas during pregnancy is a common event, has one of the lowest incidences of neural tube defects in the world? Worry about something else.

Power lines

Low frequency radiation, such as from microwaves and radio waves, has the ability to generate electrical and magnetic fields in its vicinity. Another source of these extremely low frequency effects is from high voltage power lines. Studies, many of them anecdotal and far from scientific, have linked a whole host of conditions from congenital club foot and heart disease to leukaemia in the children of parents living in close proximity to high voltage power lines. However, it is unlikely that the very weak magnetic fields generated by power lines could cause malignancy or genetic effects. The earth itself generates a magnetic field which is nowhere stronger than 67 μT (magnetism is measured in Tesla (T)). Domestic electrical appliances generate fields of between 1 μT and 30 μT under normal conditions of use. The largest power lines are unable to generate field strengths of greater than 40 μT and it seems improbable to say the least that they are able to cause damage to the baby's DNA.

SMOKING

Despite the common view that the smoking habit is on the decline, smoking by women, particularly young women, is on the increase. While some women attempt to give up or certainly to cut down before and during pregnancy, a majority do not. These smokers tend to be young and, among the heaviest smokers, poorly educated and of lower social class. Smokers may find it more difficult to get pregnant: one study reported one and a half times as many women who had never been pregnant among smokers compared to non-smokers. Smokers are more likely to have their pregnancies end in miscarriage and stillbirth. The clearest risk of maternal smoking, however, is the delivery of a low birthweight baby, with a strong relationship between the number of cigarettes smoked per day and both the incidence of babies being born prematurely and the reduction in birthweight. The average weight difference between a baby born to a smoker and a non-smoker is about 200 g. This may not seem very much but it can represent a crucial difference if the baby is born prematurely. The effect of smoking on birthweight is, it would seem, reversible; a recent study showed that the birthweight of babies born to mothers who stopped smoking after the sixteenth week of pregnancy was essentially the same as for babies born to non-smokers. Since maternal smoking is known to be a major risk factor in cot death, it is never too late to give it up.

Having said all of this, there is no sound evidence that smoking fewer than five cigarettes a day is harmful to the baby. It is also evident that the effects of smoking are potentiated by such things as alcohol intake, inadequate diet and poverty. What of handicap? There is a higher incidence of handicap among babies of shorter gestational age and low birthweight, and this type of baby is born more frequently to smokers than non-smokers. However, taken overall, a number of large-scale studies have reported no significant increase in congenital abnormalities in babies born to smokers. Perhaps the relevant statistics here are not those related to the baby at all – remember smoking 20 cigarettes a day gives you a 1 in 200 chance of dying as a result of your habit.

TERATOGENS

Teratogens are agents that adversely affect a baby that was previously developing normally, causing handicap and sometimes death. The best known teratogens include chemicals (drugs), radiation and infectious agents. Although ionizing radiation, which I have already discussed, has of course a potent teratogenic effect, the reality is that very few of us are ever likely to come into contact with the level of radiation that constitutes a severe risk to our baby. Drugs and infections, however, are a different matter.

It is important to get a grip on the principles of teratology in order to understand why a teratogen may affect one baby but not another in identical circumstances, and why a teratogen may wreak havoc at one stage of pregnancy but produce no effect at another. Teratogens have different effects in different species – for instance, thalidomide has no effect on developing rat embryos while in primates it causes the characteristic limb reductions (phocomelia) seen in victims of the thalidomide tragedy. Conversely, cortisol, a human stress hormone, is a teratogen in rodents.

The time at which a baby is exposed to a potential teratogen is of crucial importance. In the first two weeks of embryonic life, there seems to be an all–or–nothing response – either lethal or the embryo survives with no abnormality. This may be because if one cell is destroyed by the effect of the teratogen, a surviving cell may be able to assume its function since cells at this stage have not differentiated irrevocably into cells destined to become specific organs.

The process by which a ball of cells turns into a baby, complete with organ systems, occurs between the 3rd and 8th embryonic week, i.e. between the 5th and 10th menstrual week. (Embryonic weeks are two weeks behind the menstrual weeks in which pregnancy gestation is calculated because pregnancy stage is based on the first day of your last period and will therefore include two weeks when you weren't actually pregnant.) It is during this period of organogenesis that a baby is most susceptible to teratogens. Teratogens act in an organ-specific way, affecting one organ at one particular time but another at a different stage of development. The precise time at which the teratogen is introduced to the developing baby will determine not only whether a malformation occurs, but the specific spectrum of anomalies. For instance, it is known that in the rat, radiation produces no anomalies on Day 8 or Day 11, but numerous abnormalities on Day 9 (eye, brain, spinal cord, heart, aortic arch and urinary system) and also on Day 10, although these are different from those caused by exposure on Day 9 (eye, brain and urinary system).

The development of the baby's organs is complete by the 12th week of pregnancy; thereafter, the main developmental process is one of growth. Thus after this stage of pregnancy a teratogen may affect a baby's growth but will produce no visible malformations.

Not all babies react in the same way to teratogens. This is because the genetic make-up of both the mother and the baby influences the action of a teratogen. For instance, there is a well-known case in which a woman who was pregnant with non-identical twins, fathered by different men, was exposed to the anti-convulsant drug diphenylhydantoin. The twin who had been fathered by a black man was unaffected, but the one fathered by a white man developed the hydantoin syndrome (a specific range of abnormalities caused by this chemical). Since the environment in the womb and indeed the mother were identical for both twins, the difference in teratogenic effects can only be explained by genetic differences in susceptibility. Actually, this difference in susceptibility to drugs is something that you are probably already aware of. You no doubt know someone who has taken the same medicine as you have, only to suffer side-effects that you have not experienced at all. At the other extreme, some people are completely resistant to a specific drug, for instance, the anti-coagulant drug warfarin. Thus the genetic make-up of your baby will be a considerable influence as to whether or not it is affected by a teratogen.

The effect of teratogens can also be modified, with one agent promoting the potential teratogenicity of another. It is known that the food preservative benzoic acid enhances aspirin teratogenicity in rats. (Before you panic, no, aspirin is not a teratogen in humans.) Other influential factors are the weight of the baby and weight of the mother, how good the blood supply to the baby is, the position of the baby in the womb, and diet (inasmuch as diet determines maternal weight, and thus the baby's weight). Given all of this, it is no surprise to find that it is incredibly difficult to prove that a particular agent is a teratogen, not least because similar abnormalities may occur in women who were definitely not exposed to teratogens in pregnancy. Several factors can implicate a particular agent: if an anomaly or pattern of anomalies is consistently associated with a suspected teratogen, if the agent was present during the stage of pregnancy when such anomalies could plausibly have arisen, and if the anomaly was less common before the potential teratogen was available (limb defects of the type associated with thalidomide were almost unknown before the introduction of thalidomide). As we have seen, giving animals a suspected teratogen in an attempt to produce the same anomalies may be of no use at all because of the differences in teratogen susceptibilities between species.

MEDICINES AND DRUGS

If there is any health message that the British public have received loud and clear, it is that you should not take drugs in pregnancy. While in the light of thalidomide this is an important message, it has probably been overstated as women now believe that almost any drug taken in the early months of pregnancy will cause malformation. In truth, there are only a handful of drugs that are proven teratogens, including thalidomide.

Before discussing medicines at greater length, however, a word about their names. Most medicines have several names, not just their chemical name but also trade names as well. The same drug may have several different trade names, reflecting different strengths of the drug, as well as the fact that they are manufactured by different companies. A further confusion is that British trade names for one product may be quite different from the name for the same product in another country – Tylanol is the American equivalent of Panadol, for instance. Wherever possible I have given you the chemical name of the drug (which always starts with a lower-case letter) followed by the brand name or names (if there are any), which always starts with a capital letter.

Five of the known drug teratogens are anti-cancer drugs, chlorambucil, busulphan, actinomycin, mercaptopurine and methotrexate (none of which would be prescribed outside a hospital setting). Preparations likely to be prescribed only by hospital skin specialists for very severe acne, etretinate and isoretinoin which are Vitamin A derivatives, are also highly teratogenic. Advice is to defer conception for two years after etretinate and four weeks after isoretinoin. You should be reassured that no over-the-counter acne preparations contain these compounds. Sodium valproate (Epilim, used in the treatment of epilepsy) and lithium (Camcolit, Liskonum, Phasal, Priadel, used in the treatment of psychosis) should not be used in pregnancy. However, it should be said that the majority of women taking these last-named drugs will still have normal babies.

The general rule for prescribing in pregnancy is not to prescribe unless necessary and then to use only those drugs which have been in use for many years without ill effects. Because of the thalidomide tragedy and mindful of the huge costs involved should a drug prove to be teratogenic, most new drugs are not tested at all for use in pregnancy and given a blanket 'not for use in pregnancy' label. This does not mean that these drugs are known teratogens, just that they have not been tested for use in pregnancy which is quite a different thing. Some drug sheets may report evidence of animal teratogenicity. This is a warning signal that caution might be appropriate when prescribing in pregnancy, not a statement that a drug is a human teratogen.

The British National Formulary (the *BNF*) is published jointly every six months by the British Medical Association and the Royal Pharmaceutical Society of Great Britain and can be obtained from the reference section of your local library. It lists a table of drugs to be avoided or used with caution in pregnancy, not only the ones that are teratogens but also others which cross the placenta and affect the baby's metabolism or well-being. For example, the use of thiazides (diuretics, to control water balance) can in rare instances affect the baby's blood and it would therefore be better to be cautious and to use another type of diuretic.

Thus, while assuming all medicines are unsafe to take during pregnancy (and this includes over-the-counter medicines), be reassured that very few drugs are actually teratogenic and that even if they are, unless you have taken them in the appropriate time window, they may not affect your baby.

Ideally, women should avoid taking medicine at the time of conception and during the first three months. However, this assumes knowledge of pregnancy and while we might all wish that babies were planned the reality is that only 25 per cent of them actually are planned. There is therefore quite a high chance that you may inadvertently be taking a medicine for a common ailment during the early part of your pregnancy. The effects of some of these medicines are discussed below.

Antibiotics

Antibiotics are probably the drugs that are most often taken inadvertently during early pregnancy. Penicillin (many, many trade names including Amoxil, Ampicillin, etc.) and erythromycin (Erythrocin, Erycen, Erythroped) are known to be safe.

The antibiotics commonly used to treat urinary tract infections (short-acting sulphonamides such as co-trimoxazole (Septrin)) have been used widely in pregnancy without effect although there is a theoretical question mark over their use because they affect the body's use of folic acid. Chloramphenicol (Chloromycetin) is safe although it should not be used in late pregnancy because of the danger of causing the so-called 'grey syndrome' in which the baby shows signs of cardio-vascular collapse. The use of tetracycline (Achromycin, Panmycin, Tetrex, Sustamycin) in pregnancy causes permanent discoloration of the baby's teeth but no other abnormalities. The use of streptomycin (used in the treatment of TB) is associated with a small risk of deafness. There is also a theoretical question mark over the anti-TB antibiotic, rifampicin.

Analgesics

There are very few of us who do not occasionally take a couple of aspirin for a blinding headache, and this may well have inadvertently occurred during early pregnancy. Pregnant women are no different from other women – they will continue to get the odd headache during pregnancy and there is no need for them to suffer in silence for fear of harming their baby. Aspirin is not known to be a teratogen and the occasional couple of aspirin would seem to be harmless. However, large doses of aspirin in late pregnancy are associated with bleeding in the newborn and so should be avoided. Paracetamol is not a teratogen either and is the mild analgesic of choice in pregnancy. The analgesic in Nurofen (ibuprofen) also appears to be safe.

Tranquillizers

Findings fail to show any association between diazepam and congenital abnormality. Use of other minor tranquillizers in pregnancy has been studied, with results being contradictory but in general making only the very weakest of associations between tranquillizer use and subsequent abnormality.

Oral contraceptives

The debate over whether inadvertent use of oral contraceptives during pregnancy is associated with fetal abnormality has raged for many years. In 1990 a summary of all available data concluded that exposure to oral contraceptives did not increase the risk of anomalies over that in non-exposed populations.

Infertility drugs

The jury is still out on the association between specific anomalies and the use of clomiphene citrate, used to induce ovulation in women experiencing infertility problems. The number of cases of abnormality reported is minute (just 12 in the US compared to hundreds of thousands of women taking the drug) and weighed against the possibility of not having a baby at all, this risk has to be considered one worth taking.

I have discussed simply the most common drugs here. For those on long-term medication, such as anti-coagulant therapy where heparin should be used in preference to warfarin which has specific risks associated with it, you are probably already aware that there might be a possible problem in pregnancy. As I have stressed, the number of drugs that are known teratogens is in fact very small but if you are on long-term drug therapy, discuss the possible implications of your drug regime with your specialist before pregnancy.

An example of this is the drugs used in the treatment of epilepsy. There is a small risk (2 per cent) of neural tube defects associated with the use of sodium valproate (Epilim). There is a 5 per cent risk of a baby having abnormalities (usually cleft palate or heart defects) associated with the use of phenytoin sodium (Epaneutin). There is a 1 per cent risk of minor malformations associated with the use of carbamazepine (Tegratol). Switching to another drug such as phenobarbitol (no known teratogenic effect), giving folic acid supplements concurrently if phenytoin is used, not using combinations of drugs and reducing dosage to the minimum possible are all indicated, as indeed would be careful ultrasound scanning at about 16–18 weeks. For some women, it may be possible, in consultation with their specialist, to give up their medication altogether. There is no known association between congenital malformation and the occurrence of convulsions in pregnancy but epileptics as a group are known to have a two-fold increase in the risk of having an abnormal baby independent of drugs.

Asthma

The drugs used in the treatment of asthma are not known to cause damage to the baby, although the use of theophylline may have a transient effect on the condition of the baby at birth.

Anaesthetics

There is no association between anaesthetics and congenital malformations. There is, however, an association between chronic exposure (not one-off episodes of anaesthesia for surgery, etc. but working with anaesthetics on a daily basis by theatre staff and doctors) and a slightly increased rate of spontaneous miscarriage.

Recreational drugs

No evidence of marijuana teratogenicity exists, but there is no assurance that it is safe either. It is difficult to pinpoint the effects of hard drugs such as LSD, crack and cocaine whose users are from their lifestyle alone at far greater risk of numerous obstetric complications. The use of cocaine (or alkaloidal cocaine – crack) is not associated with physical abnormality although it is the cause of low birthweight, placental abruption, fetal distress, mental retardation, decreased interactive behaviour and so on – the full list is a sad and very long one.

Alcohol

One of the most significant teratogenic risks to the baby arises from alcohol use by the mother. Alcohol abuse is the most common drug abuse problem in contemporary society, affecting about 2 per cent of women of childbearing age. The Fetal Alcohol Syndrome (FAS) was first reported among children born to mothers who were alcoholic. Such babies display a characteristic range of physical malformations, including a typical flattened facial appearance, and may also have mental retardation, cardiac defects and behavioural problems. The incidence of FAS is, to be honest, unknown, with estimates ranging from 90 per 1,000 births, to 1 in 1,500 to 'very rare'. Most hospitals in Britain see at least a couple of cases a year, with some hospitals seeing more. Studies with mice showed that oral alcohol could damage newly fertilized eggs. Although some would say that stone cold sober conception is to be preferred, the reality is that a great many babies are conceived either in, or as a result of, an alcoholic haze. An ingenious piece of research in Scotland attempted to compare the outcome in babies known to be conceived over the Christmas and New Year period with babies conceived at other times of the year. They failed in their attempt but I am unaware of an increase in the incidence of handicapping conditions among babies born in September and October.

Even if the baby is conceived with both partners sober, it is still likely that a woman may have an inadvertent drink or two before recognition of pregnancy. The risk is not great, if there is any risk at all. Binge drinking at a crucial time of organogenesis is probably much more dangerous than the occasional drink on a more regular basis but if you want to know how many drinks constitutes binge drinking or what the crucial period is, you are not likely to find a consistent answer, even among experts in this field – 'We don't know' is the honest reply. Certainly even moderate drinking in pregnancy (two drinks or more a day) is associated with increased risk of miscarriage and of fetal growth retardation, although there is no such association with one drink or less a day. There is much evidence that even for the very heavy drinker, reduction of alcohol intake can reduce the incidence of growth retardation, and it is not a foregone conclusion that all alcoholics will have babies with FAS, because they don't. The sensible advice is that the odd drink will do no harm but you should try to cut out alcohol altogether throughout your pregnancy.

Vitamin A

The toxicity of Vitamin A, which is stored and concentrated in the liver, was first discovered when early polar explorers died as a result of eating polar bear liver. Polar bears, it appears, have a diet containing mega amounts of Vitamin A from constant munching on seal livers. As a result their own livers are chock full of the stuff – and highly toxic. Vitamin A is a potent teratogen and as outlined, drugs containing Vitamin A derivatives (such as those used in the treatment of acne) must not be used in pregnancy.

The notification of a case of Vitamin A damage in the baby of a woman who ate large amounts of liver led to an investigation of Vitamin A levels in the liver of livestock, which were found to be far higher than expected. It transpired that livestock were being fed on foodstuffs which were routinely supplemented with Vitamin A. The excess of Vitamin A was not being excreted (Vitamin A is not a water-soluble vitamin) but was being stored in the animals' livers. This led to the subsequent recommendation of the Department of Health that pregnant women should not eat liver at all in pregnancy and should also restrict their intake of liver-based products such as liver sausages and pâtés. If you have inadvertently eaten liver in early pregnancy, do not panic. Although it is preferable not to eat liver, the occasional plateful will not cause damage, although it will furnish you with enough Vitamin A to keep you going for months. It is worth noting that many of our foods are, in a similar way, routinely supplemented – these include cereals and also margarines which are fortified by law. Taking even quite small Vitamin A supplements can push women over the recommended daily intake level. As noted before, vitamin supplements without appropriate medical advice are not necessary and may even be harmful.

Vaccines

There is no direct evidence that vaccination with killed or attenuated live vaccines against influenza, tetanus, cholera or yellow fever is harmful to the baby. It is preferable for women not to have typhoid, polio or smallpox vaccination in pregnancy, although they have been given without ill effect. Rubella vaccination should not be given in pregnancy. However, there is actually a very low risk of fetal effects (see page 80) and of the 522 infants in the US born to mothers known to have been inadvertently immunized with rubella vaccine, none has so far developed any defects compatible with congenital rubella.

INFECTIONS

Infectious agents account for a significant proportion of congenital and developmental handicaps. Toxoplasma and cytomegalovirus (CMV), together with diagnostic and testing strategies, are discussed later in Chapter 5. Once again, the critical timing of teratogens is evident with rubella (German measles), which has little effect on the developing baby after the 16th week of pregnancy but potentially devastating effects before this time. It is important to stress that infection in the mother doesn't necessarily mean that the baby will be infected too. Also the severity of the mother's infection is not necessarily indicative of fetal infection.

Colds and flu

There is no evidence that a cold either at the time of conception or during early pregnancy causes abnormalities. The evidence on flu is less reassuring as there have been a number of studies showing an increased anomaly rate among women who had flu in pregnancy. However there are just as many studies showing no effect. High temperatures may be particularly significant in this regard and if you do have a high temperature, you should take, under your doctor's directions, fever-lowering drugs such as paracetamol at regular intervals. You should also do everything you can to allow your body to lose heat quickly, i.e. only a light bedcovering, frequent tepid baths, etc.

Chickenpox

Over 90 per cent of women are immune to chickenpox (varicella zoster virus) by the time they become pregnant. There is therefore a very high chance that you are immune, sometimes even if you don't remember having chickenpox.

But if you definitely haven't had it, when pregnant you should try to avoid contact with families in the throes of chickenpox. There is a risk – although very low (less than 5 per cent) – of severe multiple congenital anomalies if non-immune women are exposed to varicella during the first trimester. Typical anomalies are skin lesions, limb reduction, mental retardation and eye abnormalities. Of greater concern perhaps is that chickenpox contracted for the first time in pregnancy can be a very severe illness indeed with a significant number of women requiring respiratory support. If maternal infection occurs in the four days prior to delivery, life-threatening illness may develop in the baby soon after birth.

Rubella (German measles)

In the period 1970–74 the annual number of cases of congenital rubella was 69. By 1987, following the instigation of the rubella immunization programme, the annual incidence was down to 23 cases. In the USA, where admission to primary school is refused until a child has had the MMR vaccine (mumps, measles, rubella), there has been an even more dramatic fall in numbers from 62 in 1969 to just two cases in 1987. The effects of contracting rubella in the first trimester of pregnancy are well known; they are principally cataracts, malformations of the heart and deafness which ranges from severe disability to a hearing loss only detectable by audiometry.

Rubella is almost impossible to diagnose from clinical signs alone and advice is often sought by women who have been in contact with someone with rubella – usually a child – or who have developed a rash. A blood sample is taken within the first two to three days of onset of the rash. A second sample is taken about eight days later to see whether antibodies to rubella have developed. Recent infection is indicated by the presence of IgM rubella antibodies. Occasional false positive results do occur so a repeat test may be made before a definite diagnosis is made. One of the major problems of rubella infection is that 50 per cent of babies will not have been infected by rubella, even though their mothers have the infection. However, it is only possible to make this diagnosis after 21 weeks of pregnancy when the fetal immune system is more fully developed and cordocentesis can be used to obtain a fetal blood sample. Many mothers faced with the possible severity of handicap (defects such as deafness and blindness cannot be determined by ultrasound scanning) opt to terminate their pregnancies before the first trimester is over, rather than wait for further diagnosis and risk a second trimester termination. If you, or someone you know, is in this awful situation of having confirmed rubella infection in early pregnancy, without knowing whether their baby is affected, the best advice is to seek help from one of the six or so specialist fetal medicine centres in Britain listed at the back of this book.

OTHER RISKS

Much of what has been discussed in this chapter with regard to risk is rather nebulous. However, the next section deals with risk factors that statisticians can really get their teeth into. In general these are risks that cannot be changed or avoided – if you are 40, you are 40 and there's not a lot you can do about it.

Maternal age

As you get older, the risks of having a baby with chromosomal disorder increase sharply. This fact, together with a testing strategy for the older mother, is discussed more fully in Chapter 6. People often ask me whether risk of handicap also increases with paternal age. Except for one or two well-known examples, such as the type of dwarfism called achondroplasia, there is no known association between older fathers and fetal handicap.

Ethnic group

Certain ethnic groups are at risk from specific handicapping conditions, for instance, 1 in 30 Ashkenazi Jews, compared to 1 in 300 in other ethnic groups, are carriers of Tay-Sachs disease. Thalassaemia is more common in Italians (carrier frequency 1 in 50), Greeks (1 in 14) and Cypriots (1 in 6). West Indian, US and African blacks are at greatest risk from sickle-cell disease. If you fall into any of these ethnic groups, you may already have had counselling and know whether or not you are a carrier. Alternatively, you may want to have prenatal testing (the appropriate test for each of these conditions is given in the glossary).

Existing chronic medical condition

There are four main risks associated with pregnancy when you have a pre-existing chronic medical condition such as diabetes, kidney disease, epilepsy, hypertension, etc. One risk is that your own condition will either be permanently worsened by pregnancy (as may be the case with women with pre-existing kidney disease) or become temporarily worsened with possible consequences for the baby (such as with existing hypertension). Another concern is what chance your baby has of having your medical condition – for the record, the odds of an epileptic woman having a child that is epileptic are 1 in 30. As we saw earlier with the discussion on drugs in epilepsy, there is also a risk that the drugs used to treat your condition may be harmful to the baby. Finally, as with diabetes and epilepsy, there is a risk that the condition itself may adversely affect the baby. With epilepsy there is an increased risk of fetal anomaly, independent of drugs, although this is small. For diabetics, there is a risk that the baby may grow very large (macrosomia), and that the baby will have respiratory problems at birth. In the past, babies born to diabetic mothers tended to have a higher risk of anomaly, with limb defects being the most commonly seen type. However, experience has shown that immaculate control of sugar, not only during pregnancy but crucially in the period leading up to and at conception, is the key factor in the prevention of these defects. As pointed out in the chapter on tests prior to pregnancy, all women with pre-existing disease would be strongly advised to discuss with their specialist their condition and the possible impact of pregnancy before getting pregnant. Such a discussion allows a woman and her partner to understand fully her individual risks, which are not possible to quote here. Having specialist advice can also provide solid reassurance based on that specialist's wide experience of women with your type of problem who become pregnant. Measures can be taken to alter drug regimes to ones most suitable to pregnancy. It is also important to know exactly what the status of your condition is prior to pregnancy, so that baseline measurements can be obtained in order that your own condition, never mind that of the baby, can be monitored in pregnancy.

PKU

Women who had the metabolic disease phenylketoneuria (PKU) in childhood, who will have had a diet low in the amino acid phenylalanine in their early years, need to return to a special diet during pregnancy in order to reduce the chances of a baby with disability, specifically cretinism.

Previous obstetric history

A history of three or more miscarriages would indicate a need to send blood from both parents to be karyotyped prior to the next pregnancy, just to check whether a chromosome problem (a balanced translocation, explained more fully in the glossary) is the cause, although this accounts for only a small number of cases of repeated miscarriage. Intensive monitoring of pregnancy with ultrasound, on a weekly basis in the first three months, might also be suggested – more for the reassurance it gives you than for any medical reason to check on your baby's progress. If anyone in your close family has an obstetric history which includes many unexplained miscarriages or stillbirths, it is probably worth mentioning it as it may alert your doctor to the possibility of a chromosome abnormality in the family.

If you have had a previous pregnancy in which the baby was very severely growth retarded, either dying in the womb or at birth, a chromosome abnormality may have been the cause. Normally the baby is karyotyped following death and the results of such investigation may be a pointer to the management of a subsequent pregnancy. Genetic counselling may be indicated, depending on the results of the karyotype.

Finally, having had a baby with a handicap in a previous pregnancy may sharply increase the odds of having another, although the risks of recurrence of chromosomal defects such as Down's syndrome are generally small (about 1 in 100). A word about increased odds. Let us say that there is an abnormality called pink parrot. Before your first pregnancy, the odds of you having a baby with pink parrot were calculated by knowing the number of all births and putting against it the number of babies born with pink parrot. If you then have a baby with this condition, you become a member of a very exclusive club, with relatively few members. Your odds of having a second baby with it are then calculated not with the huge numbers involved in the first calculation, but with much smaller numbers. It's a bit like saying what are the odds of a woman in Britain having a sequinned ballgown: not very great. But if you gathered together all the women who did ballroom dancing and asked the same question, you'd get much reduced odds. In the same way it is possible, without you perceiving any other increase in risk factors, to be at much increased risk a second time around.

Consanguinity

If the father of the baby you are expecting is a close relative, the chances of you having a genetically abnormal baby are increased quite considerably. This may be something that you feel quite happy to discuss openly with your carers if you have married a cousin but if the relationship is a closer one, then ask to see your consultant privately and discuss it with him or her in confidence.

Family history of genetic disease

We discuss this in greater detail in Chapter 8 on genetic counselling.

Pre-pregnancy counselling

Pre-pregnancy counselling can clearly benefit women with particular health problems or those to whom previous pregnancy has brought difficulties, or where there is a history of genetic disease. Whether pre-pregnancy counselling has any significant benefit for the normal, healthy woman is debatable. In general women who are sufficiently motivated to attend a pre-pregnancy counselling clinic are middle class. Their health is better than that of their working-class sisters, and they eat better, exercise more and smoke and drink less. As a result, they are much more likely to have a healthy baby and to have already taken up activities which promote good health. Attendance at such a clinic implies that these women believe that every aspect of conception, pregnancy and birth can be managed in order to produce a perfect baby. But it remains true to say that most pregnancy complications are unpredictable or can only be managed in the crudest way, for instance by early delivery of the baby in a mother who has pre-eclampsia. When things go wrong, a woman may then believe that it is her fault. Pre-pregnancy counselling can be very guilt-inducing for, if a woman ignores the advice given – for instance, not to smoke – she may continue to feel guilty and inadequate throughout her pregnancy. It is all very well to take the moral high ground and say every woman should think about potential risks to her baby before and during the time she is pregnant and do everything to avoid them, but real life just ain't like that. Much risk is simply unavoidable and sometimes, just like lightning in St Albans, we just have to go out and get on with it – putting risk into its proper place as we do so.

4   Ultrasound

Ultrasound is familiar to almost all pregnant women, yet its limitations as regards antenatal diagnosis are not understood.

Background If you've ever watched one of those interminable destroyers versus U-boat films on television on a wet afternoon, then you have seen the principles of ultrasound at work. There is not much difference between looking for a submarine in the North Sea and looking for a baby in a pool of amniotic fluid; the theory behind it – that of echo location of an object – is the same, even if the scale of operation is somewhat smaller. Professor Ian Donald was the remarkable man who first applied the techniques of ultrasound to pregnancy. At the time, in the middle 1950s, people thought he was barking mad. The equipment was bulky in the extreme – early pictures show a room full of equipment with a pregnant mother squashed into one small corner. Today over 90 per cent of pregnant women have an ultrasound scan during pregnancy and ultrasound has revolutionized obstetrics.

During an ultrasound scan sound waves are emitted from a small hand-held device called a transducer. As the transducer is moved over the mother's abdomen, the sound waves are reflected back as echoes. The echoes (now in the form of electrical signals) are received by the transducer and transmitted to a computer which uses the signals to build up a two-dimensional black and white picture which appears on a television screen. The echoes are reflected in different ways depending on the type of tissue that they encounter and are bounced back by. Thus it is that you can distinguish between bone, tissue and fluid. By combining a series of still pictures in rapid succession, movement can be seen – rather in the same way that you can flick the pages of some comic books and see a figure move. This is called real time ultrasound.

Quality of ultrasound equipment is, in general, less important than the skills of the operator. The skill comes from interpreting what are two-dimensional pictures in a three-dimensional way and from avoiding incorrect interpretations due to artefacts, that is structures that appear to be present but which in reality are simply produced by confusions in the echo pattern.

Doppler ultrasound

A different method of using ultrasound to give information about the baby has been developed over the last few years. This is called Doppler ultrasound. You might like to think of this as being a machine which, although it works on the same principles as ordinary ultrasound, generates noise rather than pictures. This noise is translated on a television screen into a wave pattern rather than an image. You may dimly remember something about Doppler from your schooldays. In fact, most of us unwittingly come across the Doppler effect on a regular basis. For instance, as a police car with a wailing siren comes screeching down the road towards you, the note of the siren seems to change as the car passes you – the Doppler effect. And the change in sound is called the Doppler shift. By bouncing sound off blood cells as they rush through blood vessels and noting the Doppler shift, the speed and therefore the amount of blood flow can be determined. The principal use of this type of ultrasound is to track blood flow through different blood vessels in the baby, and thus directly to assess the baby's state of health. Some of the newest Doppler machines incorporate colour, so that venous blood flow comes up blue on the screen and arterial blood flow appears as red. Poor Doppler blood flow patterns in the umbilical vessels in

otherwise seemingly healthy babies have been linked to undetected chromosome abnormality, small for dates babies (that
is, babies that are smaller than they should be for their
gestational age) and possible unexplained stillbirth. However,
large-scale studies of the use of Doppler ultrasound as a
screening device have failed to show any conclusive benefits.
But Doppler scans are of very considerable benefit to women
with high risk pregnancies and you will find them in use in
teaching hospitals.

Levels of ultrasound

To most women, ultrasound is ultrasound and all scans appear
to be very much the same. Actually, leaving aside Doppler
ultrasound, there are three quite distinct levels of obstetric
ultrasound and it's important to know which you are having,
if you are to understand the limitations of the process. Basic
real-time ultrasound is usually undertaken by technicians
rather than doctors. You may find that it is also used by
midwives or GPs in non-hospital settings. The scan will last
for no more than five or at most ten minutes. It is used simply
to see whether there is a baby there, how big it is and whether
there is more than one baby. Only the most severe of
malformations could be seen using this type of scanning
procedure. It is unlikely that the operators of this level of scan
have sufficient skills to interpret what they see with any
accuracy. This type of scan would not constitute a screen for
physical malformation in your baby.

Level 2 'fetal anomaly scanning' is suitable for screening for
abnormality and is the sort of scanning that most women are
likely to receive in a big general hospital. It will take between
15 and 20 minutes to perform, and will be carried out by
someone specially trained in the use of ultrasound. It will
usually be undertaken in hospital either in or close to the

maternity unit. The operator will scan your baby, using a checklist to make sure that he or she has covered everything. This type of scanning would be used in conjunction with amniocentesis.

Level 3 scanning is of a very high quality and is offered at specialist centres only, usually teaching hospitals. The operator will be a doctor, usually with considerable expertise. Such an operator would be able to observe the baby both in the first and second trimester of pregnancy, be able to assess fetal movements and diagnose fetal abnormalities with a high degree of accuracy. This type of ultrasound is used in conjunction with CVS (page 113), with fetal blood sampling and with fetal treatments such as transfusion.

Because ultrasound is associated with scanning for fetal abnormality, women tend to forget that it has a host of other uses. We shall briefly consider these so that you understand what each scan you have is for. If you are having a scan for any of these reasons below, particularly in connection with threatened miscarriage, location of placenta, etc., your baby is not necessarily being checked for abnormality as well. In other words, ultrasound scanning is very much a question of horses for courses; the level of scanning that you have, in terms of expertise rather than equipment, is all.

Assessing your baby's well being

It may sound blindingly obvious, but one of the main uses of ultrasound is to see whether there is a baby in the womb and whether its heart is still beating. This is particularly important for women who have been experiencing bleeding or pain in early pregnancy, women in whom ectopic pregnancy is suspected, or for women who, having had a positive pregnancy test, have stopped feeling pregnant (indicating the type of miscarriage known as a missed abortion). Given that 50 per cent of women who threaten to miscarry in early pregnancy go on to have a normal full term baby, the reassurance that ultrasound provides in demonstrating that the baby is not only still there, but looks fine, cannot be underestimated. Needless to say, if there is more than one baby then ultrasound will show this.

Determining where the placenta is located

The source of bleeding in later pregnancy can often be pinpointed with ultrasound and the location, size and structure of the placenta assessed. This is important in deciding method of delivery for those women who have placenta praevia – a placenta that covers the cervix, either partially or totally. One word on this. True placenta praevia is usually confirmed with ultrasound following an episode of light, intermittent bleeding (vaginal spotting) and there is no other option but to deliver the baby by Caesarean section. However, many women are told that they have a low-lying placenta when having a routine dating scan. They are then told not to worry and that the placenta will probably move, which leads to great confusion because most women are quite rightly of the opinion that the placenta is firmly fixed in one spot. What actually happens is that as the womb grows so the placenta is pulled up, away from the cervix. In the majority of cases, a scan a few weeks later reveals that there is no longer a problem.

Assessing your baby's age and rate of growth

If you are unsure of the date of your last period or when you conceived, ultrasound can be used to date your pregnancy and give you a better estimate of your date of delivery. Dating of pregnancy can be fairly accurate in early pregnancy, usually to within a week either side, which is as good as you get with a certain date of last period, but after about 22 weeks it becomes far less reliable and there is a much bigger margin of error. A number of measurements are made. These include the length of the baby's leg bone, the diameter of the head and the abdominal circumference. These are then compared to standard 'growth charts' which will show what gestation the measurements indicate. Dating your pregnancy accurately is not just about knowing your due delivery date. The results of screening tests such as triple test become inaccurate if they are based on an incorrect assessment of gestational age, thus ultrasound screening is likely to become even more important.

The record of your baby's vital statistics at a certain age of pregnancy may sit in your file and, apart from dating your pregnancy, may be of no further use. However, if for some reason it is thought that your baby is not thriving, then these measurements come into their own, as they will show whether your baby's development has slowed down, or even halted, from the baseline of measurements established in early pregnancy.

Determination of fetal sex

Can you, can't you? People with lots of experience claim to be able to tell the sex of a baby from an ultrasound scan – be warned, they can be wrong. There's nothing so confusing as all those loops of umbilical cord between the legs. If fetal sex really matters, karyotyping is the only way to be certain.

HAVING AN ULTRASOUND SCAN

Unless the hospital you are booked with has a vaginal ultrasound machine (where the transducer sits in the vagina, rather than being slid over the abdomen), a full bladder is required in order to get the best picture of your baby in the early months of pregnancy. Later on, a good picture is possible without a full bladder. You will be asked to drink a set amount (usually a couple of pints) an hour or so before the scan is due.

You will be asked to lie flat on a table, and to hitch up your skirt above your navel. You will be asked to take your tights off but to leave your knickers on. Some mineral oil or special ultrasound jelly will then be smeared on your lower abdomen so that the transducer glides easily across it. The lights will then be dimmed (to get a better view of the ultrasound screen). The transducer may have to be moved around quite a bit before the operator is satisfied with the view that he or she has obtained. Various measurements are taken. This is done automatically by the machine, sometimes in conjunction with a light pen that is moved across the screen. Some units have polaroid cameras attached to their machines and may take a picture for you of your baby. The pictures usually have the date and your name or hospital number on them – once again, this is an automatic function in most machines. Some units may ask you to pay for the picture.

Practicalities Take a spare pair of knickers with you. No matter how careful the operators are, the ultrasound jelly tends to get everywhere. Expect a bit of a frisson when the jelly goes on – it's usually freezing cold. Wear either a loose-fitting dress that you can hitch up easily or for preference wear separates.

Having a full bladder can be incredibly uncomfortable, particularly if your appointment is delayed by the length of the queue. And it doesn't help that once you have a bladder full to bursting, someone comes and leans a transducer on it! If you really are bursting, don't be afraid to tell someone and ask whether you can visit the loo, in order to wee a small amount and thus relieve the pressure. Whatever you do, don't empty your bladder completely as you will then have to sit there and be fed glasses of water until your bladder is full again.

You don't have to have your partner with you, but as an ultrasound scan is usually the first glimpse that you get of your baby, it can be a special time that you might enjoy sharing.

Risks

The National Institute of Health in America has said that, in the light of all available evidence, 'diagnostic ultrasound is considered to be a low risk procedure. However, routine use of ultrasound in pregnancy should be discouraged.' On the other hand a working party of the Royal College of Obstetricians and Gynaecologists concluded in 1984 that there was no evidence for a harmful physical effect of ultrasound. What are ordinary women to make of this? In practical terms, what it means is this. If you have a specific pregnancy problem, ultrasound can be of immense value, giving immediate answers on which to base the care of you and your baby. Even if there were long term effects of ultrasound (and short term effects have failed to be demonstrated at the levels of power used by most hospitals), these are probably as nothing in comparison to the problems faced by your baby right now. The trouble with ultrasound is that it is sometimes used instead of practical skills, rather than as an adjunct to them. You don't really need ultrasound to tell you whether you're pregnant or whether there is a multiple pregnancy – most obstetricians and midwives should be able to do this. In my view the real dangers of ultrasound are its use in inexperienced hands. We have already seen that ultrasound artefacts are there to confuse the unwary. You may receive the wrong information, making you incredibly anxious, or worse still a misdiagnosis especially with Level 1 or 2 scanning. If you are having this type of scanning and an abnormality is suspected, you can always ask to be referred to a regional centre for a second opinion. On the positive side, scanning can be the first time that women bond to their babies, and according to some studies women who have seen their babies on scan are much more likely to take notice of health advice during pregnancy, such as to give up smoking.

Diagnosis of abnormality

Here we are talking about the diagnosis of physical abnormalities which can encompass everything from external physical problems, say an extra finger, to internal structural defects, like a missing chamber to the heart. There are three main ways of spotting these: by direct visualization, for instance, not being able to see the back of the skull in a baby with anencephaly; by showing that some part of the baby has developed in a disproportionate way, for example, short limbs in cases of dwarfism; and by looking at the effect that an anomaly may have on another structure in the body – lack of amniotic fluid for instance may indicate a kidney or gut problem.

Just what can be seen with an ultrasound scan? This question is not an easy one to answer. Leaving aside the skill of the operator and the quality of the ultrasound machine, many people imagine that looking at a baby with a scan is rather like looking at a naked man through a keyhole – you just assume that you'll be able to see everything. In fact, it's not like this. For a start, what you see of your naked man depends on how he is standing – if he has his arm across his stomach you might not spot that he has a ruby in his navel, for instance. If he has his back towards you, you get an ace view of the rear but not of the front. The same strictures apply to babies in the womb who can be downright awkward and uncooperative when it comes to posing for a scan – the technical name for this is poor fetal lie. In addition, what you see depends to some extent on the mother. If the mother is very overweight, you may not get as good a view of the baby as you would like.

What you see also depends on when you look. It would be

nice to think that one detailed ultrasound scan early in pregnancy could allay all one's fears about major abnormality. While it is true that some of the gravest handicapping conditions, such as anencephaly, can be picked up as early as 10–12 weeks, many of the more common handicapping conditions cannot be spotted this early. It is thought that even with expert scan operators, only some 40 per cent of anomalies can be picked up at 20 weeks, which is the preferred gestation for a fetal anomaly scan. The figure sinks to just 15 per cent at 16 weeks. About 30 per cent of abnormalities will remain completely undetected until well after birth. Many of these are problems which may develop relatively late in pregnancy – some of the renal abnormalities, for instance, cannot be seen until about 30 weeks, when other problems, such as a small amount of amniotic fluid, may start to ring warning bells.

So what should you be able to exclude following a detailed anomaly scan? Figure 6a is a list of the structures that should be visible by ultrasound scanning by 20 weeks gestation.

Figure 6a   Structures that should be visible on ultrasound scanning by 20 weeks gestation*

HEAD	Cerebral ventricles
	Ventricular hemispheric ratio
	Cerebellum
	Choroid plexus
FACE AND NECK	Lips, palate, nose, chin
	Orbits of the eyes
	Nuchal thickening (webbing on neck)
SPINE	Longitudinal and transverse section
CHEST	Heart size, shape, four-chamber view, outflow tracts
	Pleural cavities, chest shape
	Diaphragm

ABDOMEN   Stomach
                                Outline of kidneys, genitals, bladder
                                Umbilical cord, wall of abdomen

LIMBS   Arms, legs, hands, feet

* This and following figure taken from 'Routine fetal anomaly screening', in *Antenatal Diagnosis of Fetal Abnormalities*, eds. J. O. Drife and D. Donnai, Springer Verlag 1991.

But for the reasons we have already outlined not all these features will be seen in every case, every time. In Figure 6b, which is compiled from a series of over 2,000 pregnancies, you will see how often it was possible to gain clear views of certain organs. You can see that some structures are almost always seen, while others, such as a four-chamber heart view, were observed in only 30–40 per cent of cases. Doing the scan at the right time (which may mean doing it later for over-weight mothers) and asking mothers to come back if the heart can't be seen dramatically improves the rate of four-chamber observation.

Figure 6b   Visualization of organs

Organ	% visualized
HEAD	93–94
HEART	30–33
STOMACH	92–97
KIDNEYS	80–87
BLADDER	80–100
DIAPHRAGM	70–80
SPINE	70–83
FINGERS & TOES	80–93

The most common congenital malformation is that of the cardiovascular system (the heart and its surrounding blood vessels), followed by abnormalities of the head and spine (in the main, neural tube defects). Routine anomaly scanning will detect two major instances of heart abnormality in every 1,000 babies scanned. More detailed scanning at a specialist centre (which may be prompted by family history) will pick up 4–5 forms of major heart disease per 1,000 patients scanned. The actual rate of heart abnormality at birth is 8 in every 1,000, although some of these will be minor defects.

One of the ways in which ultrasound diagnosis is being made more accurate is by specialist training of operators in which, instead of looking for a specific abnormality, they look for easily recognized signs instead. An example is in neural tube defects (NTDs). Small spinal lesions are actually very difficult to spot. However, babies with NTDs tend to have a banana shape to the cerebellum, the part of the brain involved in co-ordination of movement. Before 23 weeks of pregnancy, there is also a characteristic 'lemon' shape to the head (the result of a partial collapse of the skull's frontal bones). This finding is present in nearly 99 per cent of babies in the mid-trimester who have open spina bifida.

Getting results

If the person doing your ultrasound is a technician rather than an ultrasound specialist, they may not have either the authorization or the knowledge to tell you if there's anything wrong. If you are being scanned by an obstetrician, you may prefer to say to him or her before the scan that if there is a marginal problem that he or she thinks will resolve spontaneously, then you don't want to know about it. Otherwise there is a danger of acute anxiety over something that doesn't amount to anything in real terms.

If a technician undertaking the scan suspects an anomaly they may tell you of their concern, without being specific, and arrange for a definitive scan, usually within the next 48 hours.

Remember, asking you to come back again doesn't mean that there is something awful, they may simply not have seen what they wanted to see.

If on a second ultrasound a major abnormality is confirmed, it may then be suggested that you have cordocentesis to establish the baby's karyotype. This may seem unnecessary to you, especially if the malformation has already been explained to be a lethal one. Actually, it's vitally important. Sometimes a physical abnormality may be just a visible external sign of a much more extensive chromosomal problem – and counselling for your future pregnancies is dependent on having the right diagnosis of the problem in this pregnancy.

Karyotyping may also be advised in cases where there is only a small malformation. Although chromosome abnormalities such as Down's syndrome cannot be 'seen' on scan, there may be a series of physical markers which can point strongly towards Down's. The most important of these are the so-called 'nuchal folds' – thickened areas of skin around the neck which show as a darkened line on the scanning screen from about 10 weeks. There are other such markers associated with Down's, such as relatively short long bones, a gap between the big toe and the second toe and so on. It may well be that in the future, because of the problems associated with triple test (see page 138), ultrasound screening for Down's using these markers will be adopted as a screening measure rather than blood tests. Of course, ultrasound cannot provide a definitive diagnosis for Down's syndrome or any other chromosomal abnormality and if these markers were found, confirmation of karyotype would still be required. If markers were found indicating a likelihood of Down's (or other conditions) rapid karyotyping, such as that provided via cordocentesis, would be indicated.

A type of cyst in the brain area, known as a choroid plexus cyst, has a favourable outcome if it is not associated with a chromosome abnormality. If your baby has something like a choroid plexus cyst which can if not associated with a chromosome abnormality resolve itself, you will have to wait for a repeat scan, usually some weeks later, to find out what's going on. This waiting can be difficult but there isn't another way of managing this situation as yet.

Overview

Ultrasound is used throughout pregnancy for many reasons. It is capable of picking up many, but by no means all, congenital malformations. It can also point to associated chromosome disorders. It can establish a bond between you and your baby but despite the importance of this, ultrasound should be restricted to diagnosis.

5   Obtaining fetal cells for testing

To look at a baby's chromosomes, you need to obtain some of its cells. There are several ways to obtain such cells, the most familiar of which is amniocentesis which we discuss in this chapter. But there are also two other methods, chorionic villus sampling and fetal blood sampling (cordocentesis). The important thing to remember is that these are not tests in themselves – that comes later, when cells have been obtained – these are just different ways of obtaining the material for testing.

Unlike blood tests, however, these procedures are not risk free. They all carry a risk of spontaneous miscarriage. You will also need to weigh up carefully your reasons for wanting these tests and whether you are prepared to take the risks that are attached to them, in addition of course to the anxiety of waiting for results that all tests engender.

The first and best known of these procedures, amniocentesis, involves putting a hollow needle through a pregnant woman's abdomen and into her womb to remove a sample of the amniotic fluid surrounding her baby.

Background   During pregnancy, a baby luxuriates in its own private pond. The pond is enclosed within a sac made of a remarkable material called amnion which is stretchy, waterproof and very, very strong. At the beginning of pregnancy, it is the cells that line the amniotic sac which make the fluid, but at about 12 weeks of pregnancy the baby takes over, gulping the fluid down and then weeing it, making a little more along the way as it does so. Thus amniotic fluid consists pretty much of constantly recycled baby's wee.

Amniotic fluid has several important properties which make

it immensely useful in prenatal diagnosis. First, because the fluid is constantly recycled by the baby, it contains chemicals which reflect the baby's state of health – such as increased levels of alphafetoprotein (AFP) if there is a neural tube defect (see page 132). Secondly, because the baby is constantly wriggling about, cells get rubbed off its skin – in the same way that our skin cells rub off when we're washing ourselves in the bath – and these living cells then float about in the amniotic fluid. If you take a sample of amniotic fluid, you are almost bound to find some of the baby's cells floating in it.

There are too few cells initially for reliable testing to be undertaken on them, so the sample is sent to a cytogenetics laboratory for culturing. The cells are placed in a special liquid which enhances their growth. After about two weeks (although it can be longer as cells do not always grow at the same rate), the cells are taken out of the fluid and the chromosomes within the cells are studied under a microscope, or the genetic material is used for whatever other tests are thought necessary.

Sometimes it is not the baby's cells that are of interest but the amniotic fluid itself and the levels of chemicals that it contains – for instance, following a high raised serum AFP result. Late in pregnancy, samples of the amniotic fluid may be taken in order to assess the maturity of the baby's lungs. The theory behind this is that the baby's lungs secrete a fatty substance, called surfactant, which finds its way into the amniotic fluid. The ratio of two constituents of this fatty secretion, lecithin and sphingomyelin, is about 1:1 until the lungs mature, when the amount of lecithin dramatically increases. A baby with a lecithin/sphingomyelin ratio (LSR) of 2:1 is unlikely to suffer from breathing difficulties at birth and can safely be delivered early if other problems indicate the need for early delivery. If the ratio is less, then an injection of steroids (cortisone) may be given to the mother in order to hasten fetal lung development. However, this procedure is not

now as common as it once was, thanks to the improved care of premature and tiny babies at birth.

The following discussion relates principally to those amniocenteses undertaken in mid-pregnancy for fetal diagnosis, rather than amniocenteses undertaken to assess the fluid for lung maturity close to delivery.

6   Amniocentesis

In general (but see the section on early amniocentesis, page 109), amnios for fetal karyotyping are undertaken between 16 and 18 weeks of pregnancy.

You will be asked to lie flat on a bed. Depending on the type of ultrasound being used, you may need to have a full bladder (see page 93). An obstetrician will then use ultrasound to look at your baby. This is a vital first step because she or he needs to know how the baby is lying, whether you are carrying more than one baby and also if there is anything special about your pregnancy that means taking extra care (such as an awkwardly placed placenta). Your tummy will then be swabbed with antiseptic. A local anaesthetic may be injected near to the planned site of needle insertion, but often women find this more painful than the amnio itself and many hospitals prefer not to do this. Most women say that having an amnio does not hurt, particularly if they were able to relax while it was being done. You may feel that relaxation is impossible and that you would prefer to have a local anaesthetic. If this is the case, don't be shy about discussing it with your obstetrician. Most obstetricians will make sure that you can see the ultrasound screen while you are having the amnio and actually this helps, especially if you'd rather not be seeing the needle go in.

Using the ultrasound picture as a guide, the obstetrician will then push a long fine hollow needle, about four inches in length, through the abdomen and into a free pool of amniotic fluid, without touching either the baby or the placenta. Between 10 and 20 ml of fluid (about four teaspoonsful at most) is withdrawn into a syringe. Usually the fluid is clear and odourless, although it may have a faint yellowish tinge.

The yellow coloration is caused by a pigment called bilirubin which is a by-product of red blood cell destruction. Don't panic if it's bloodstained – it simply means that in inserting the needle one of your little blood vessels was punctured, in much the same way as when you blow your nose a bit hard you may get a spot of blood in your hanky. About 10 per cent of samples are bloodstained. The needle usually has a special little gadget attached to it in order to prevent your cells getting into the sample as the needle is pushed through the wall of your abdomen.

Sometimes more than one needle insertion is needed in order to collect enough fluid. A fresh needle needs to be used each time. Nobody wants to come back and have another amnio, and it's tempting for both woman and obstetrician to press on, but if no fluid or not enough fluid has been obtained by the second attempt, it's better that the obstetrician should give up and ask you to come back a week later rather than continue. This is because there is evidence that the spontaneous miscarriage rate increases with the number of attempted insertions of the needle. Almost invariably, however, enough fluid is obtained first time around at the next attempt.

If you have a rhesus negative blood group, you will be given an injection of anti-D following the amnio, just in case some of the baby's blood cells may have escaped into your circulation. In addition, if you are Rh negative, you may have a blood test before and then 20 minutes after the procedure, just to make sure that you don't need an extra anti-D injection because more fetal blood cells than anticipated have entered your bloodstream following the amnio.

After the needle has been withdrawn, a sticking plaster or small bandage will be placed over the site of needle entry. The baby will be observed again on ultrasound. The amount of fluid taken, less than 10 per cent of the total volume, will quickly be replaced by the baby, usually within a few hours, just as our blood is replaced when we donate a pint.

Practicalities Don't wear a dress as otherwise you'll end up having to strip off completely – for preference wear a loose-fitting T-shirt and a skirt or trousers. Take a clean pair of knickers in case the pair that you're wearing get covered in the jelly used with ultrasound. Take something diverting and cheery to read in case you have to wait. This is not the time for Proust.

You might like to have someone with you when you have your amnio. You'll need to explain what is involved to him or her. It's not unknown for the pregnant woman to be fine while her source of moral support is out cold on the floor after seeing the size of the needle involved. The thought of the needle is much worse than the actual procedure and many women find that the time when they need their hand held is immediately before rather than during the amnio. It's probably advisable to have someone to take you home as you may feel a bit wobbly – not because of the procedure itself, but from the sheer relief of it all being over. It's rather like any potentially stressful experience – the anticipation is sometimes worse than the actual event.

Opinions differ about how much women should rest following an amnio. Your doctor may give you specific instructions. If he or she doesn't, ask what is appropriate in your case. Try to organize your life so that you do not have to rush off to the supermarket on the day of the procedure. It will do you no harm to spend the rest of the day either with your feet up or in bed, and a week or so of taking life easy thereafter will similarly do you no harm. If you were to have a miscarriage and you had been rushing round, you'd be consumed with guilt that it was somehow your fault. It's unlikely to have been your fault, but here's one source of heartache that you can actively do something to avoid – so do it.

After your amnio, you should be alert for any rise in temperature or general feeling of being unwell and report it immediately as it might indicate an infection. The puncture wound may bleed or even leak fluid for a short while after the procedure, although the bandage should be sufficient to prevent this. If it does continue to leak it means that the hole made in the amniotic sac which normally closes up very quickly has not yet shut. Do not take off the bandage in this instance, but ring the hospital and tell them. Whatever you do, do not leak in silence – tell someone as early treatment with antibiotics is essential. Finally, if you have vaginal bleeding or spotting following an amnio, tell the hospital but don't assume that it means you are about to miscarry. It's probably just that a little blood vessel has been caught by the needle.

Problems

Complete failure to culture the cells obtained occurs following one in every hundred procedures. The reasons for this may be varied. Not enough fluid may have been obtained or something may have gone wrong in the laboratory culture. If you are told that there has been a culture failure, it does not mean that your baby has a handicap; it simply means that the cells haven't grown sufficiently to be able to carry out proper tests. If this occurs, you may be offered a further amnio. However, at this stage of your pregnancy, you might prefer to opt for fetal blood sampling (see page 122) as you will get a faster result.

Another problem which may occur is that of maternal cell contamination of the sample. As you will have seen above, every effort is made to try to avoid this. But if some of the mother's cells are in the sample it can be very tricky to be accurate about whose cells are which, especially if the baby is a girl. It's rare – only 1 in 600 cases – but it does happen, in which case you may need either to repeat the amnio or to opt for fetal blood sampling.

Finally, in a very small proportion of cases, the chromosome content of the cells does not remain true as they grow and a slightly different chromosome configuration may be found. This is an artificially created situation and it's called pseudo-mosaicism. Once again, if this happens, you may have to repeat or go for fetal blood sampling.

If you are carrying twins, there are special difficulties in ensuring that the same sac isn't sampled twice. Your obstetrician will be well aware of this potential problem and will take special care, often putting a harmless dye into the fluid that's already been sampled so it's not taken again.

Risks

The main risk to the baby is that of spontaneous miscarriage following the procedure. Risk varies with both the skill of the person doing the amniocentesis and with the individual pregnant woman. Overall, the risk of the procedure alone is probably between 0.5 and 1 per cent, that is, between 1 in 100 and 1 in 200 women having an amnio will miscarry their babies just because they had an amniocentesis during their pregnancy. But remember that 4 out of every 100 women aged between 35 and 39 are likely to miscarry anyway, whether they go for amnios or not. And if a woman is having an amnio because of suspected abnormality, a miscarriage may occur because of the problem pregnancy, not because of the amnio – although it may occur at about the same time.

The question most women want answered is, 'If I miscarry after the amnio when will it happen?' The implication that there is somehow a danger period, and that when this is passed miscarriage is no longer something to worry about, is a dangerous one. Unfortunately there is no simple answer to this question as potentially you could miscarry at any stage of pregnancy, whether or not you had an amniocentesis. The thing to hang on to is that amniocentesis is a low risk procedure and that the odds against having a miscarriage because of it are very heavily stacked in your favour.

The skill of the operator is an important factor in the safety of these procedures. For this reason, you may opt to have your amnio in a hospital where they are carried out on a regular basis. It is reasonable to ask the obstetrician how many amnios he or she does each year; anything more than 50 a year would indicate the degree of skill that comes with frequent practice.

Many women having an amniocentesis worry that the baby will be harmed by the needle. In fact this is an incredibly rare occurrence. For a start, very few amnios these days are carried out 'blind' – the vast majority of obstetricians use ultrasound to guide the needle and can 'see' where the baby is. And even on occasions when the baby has been pricked by the needle, no lasting harm has been done.

One other potential hazard to the baby is worth mentioning. Several studies have shown that there is an increase of about 1 per cent in severe unexplained breathing problems at birth in babies born to mothers who had amniocentesis during their pregnancies. Amniotic fluid plays an important part in the development of the unborn baby's lungs and early disruption in the supply of fluid may be the cause of this problem. This condition is amenable to treatment, and overall relatively few babies get this type of breathing difficulty, so it's something to bear in mind but not to worry about.

Early amniocentesis

Several centres, notably King's College Hospital in London, are experimenting with earlier amniocentesis. This is usually undertaken at about ten weeks of pregnancy. Although the number of such procedures undertaken is still relatively small, it would appear that this type of amniocentesis has a spontaneous miscarriage rate of about 1 per cent – no higher than that carried out in later pregnancy. Obviously the great advantage of it is that results are available more quickly, usually by about 14 weeks. However, there are some specific problems to be overcome. The first has to do with taking a sample from a smaller volume of fluid. After all, if you take a cup of fluid from a bucketful, you would hardly notice the change in level. Taking a cupful from a bucket that was only half full is much more noticeable. Knowing of the possible breathing problems caused by amniocentesis in later pregnancy, will early amniocentesis result in a greater incidence of lung problems in babies? The plain answer at the moment is it appears not, but no one can be categoric at this stage. A further problem has to do with the type of cells that are found in amniotic fluid at this early stage of pregnancy and the possibility that chromosome analysis might not be as accurate as a result.

Another procedure that a few women will come across is called amnifiltration. Basically this is a variation on early amniocentesis in which the fluid is withdrawn, filtered in order to separate the baby's cells and then returned to the amniotic cavity in one continuous procedure. It remains to be seen whether this procedure will be generally adopted.

Getting the results

Normally amniocentesis results take at least three weeks to come through, and sometimes as long as five weeks. It depends on the individual laboratory and also on the time that your baby's cells have taken to grow. Ask the hospital how you are likely to be notified and whether there is someone whom you can phone for results so that you can have them more quickly. Remember that the person you phone for results is unlikely to be able to interpret the findings – so ask who you should get in touch with at the hospital if there is any query on the results.

What amniocentesis results can and can't tell you. As we saw in our second chapter, testing is no guarantee of a perfect baby. If you have amniocentesis (or for that matter, CVS or cordocentesis) and cells are obtained and then karyotyping is undertaken (where the chromosomes are spread out and then counted and assessed), you can answer the question are there the right number of chromosomes here – that is, 22 pairs of autosomes and one pair of sex chromosomes. If there are, then Down's (which is caused by an additional chromosome) can be discounted with some degree of confidence. You can look at the size and shape of the chromosomes and ask are they normal. If they are, chances are (but one says this with less confidence) that the baby has a normal chromosome pattern. You can also tell whether the chromosomes come from a baby girl or a baby boy. But that's about it. There are of course 5,000 known single gene defects, many of which can be detected by prenatal diagnosis. But you can't pose 5,000 questions every time you're faced by a cell culture following amniocentesis. If there was something in a family history to make you suspect that it was worth asking one of those 5,000 questions, it would be worth doing that particular test. But while you can exclude gross chromosome abnormality by having a 'normal' amnio result, you may still have a baby who has one of those 5,000 single gene defects, or a baby with a hitherto unsuspected physical abnormality such as a heart problem.

Overview

Early amniocentesis will become increasingly important and may overtake CVS (page 113) as a method of choice for those with a history of genetic abnormality in the family but it still remains an experimental technique. Important questions about its long term implications for babies' lung development have still to be answered and culture of cells remains difficult, with a small element of error. Later amniocentesis is the safest of the surgical ways of obtaining fetal cells for testing but its principal disadvantage is that you may be 21 weeks pregnant or more before you get the result. Older mothers may prefer to avoid amniocentesis altogether and follow a regime of detailed ultrasound scans together with biochemical testing (see page 129).

7 Chorionic villus sampling

Amniocentesis has one great disadvantage – at present it cannot be undertaken until at least 12 weeks of pregnancy, with most amniocenteses being done at around 16–20 weeks. And because only a few cells can be obtained in this way, there is an additional three to five weeks wait while enough cells are cultured to make the tests reliable. The plight of women who had as much as a 50:50 chance of having a handicapped child and their weeks of worry before the results of their tests following amniocentesis came through led to the development of a technique called variously placental biopsy, chorion biopsy or, most commonly, chorionic villus sampling – CVS for short.

Background The chorion is a sort of double envelope of cells that surrounds the fertilized egg in its earliest stages. The chorion is covered in tiny little finger-like projections, called villi (from the Latin for a finger). At this stage of development, think of the baby as being enclosed in a ball which looks as if it is covered with soft branching fronds, about 200 in all, which each look a bit like a small tree. When the fertilized egg gets into the womb, the fronds on one side of the ball attach themselves to the lining of the womb. These fronds then grow like mad, forming a fluffy mass, most of which implants into the womb lining, so forming the placenta. Meanwhile, the remainder of the fronds, which are floating free, gradually recede so that at 12 weeks of pregnancy the remaining surface of the ball is smooth.

When CVS first started, it involved taking one of the floating fronds. However, sampling from the site of the placenta proved to be better, partly because there was no need to puncture the amniotic sac. If this isn't quite clear to you, think of these placental fronds as being outside the sac in the same way that the mouthpiece of a balloon is outside the balloon itself. Another reason for not taking one of the free-floating villi was that as these villi were in the process of degenerating, they might not reflect the genetic make-up of the baby.

Because the villi are made of many living cells which are of the baby's tissue type, there is, in theory, no need to culture them and almost immediate analysis is possible. However, in practice this has not proved to be the case because of concerns about accuracy, and samples are usually cultured as well. In practice then it is usually at least a week, and sometimes two, before results are available.

There are two methods of obtaining samples of chorionic villi, through the cervix and through the abdomen. Both are described here although transabdominal CVS is much the most common technique in Britain. In Italy, by comparison, almost all CVS is transcervical. CVS is a technique which requires specialist skills and, in Britain at least, you would not normally find CVS offered outside the context of a big teaching hospital.

How and when the test is done

Chorionic villus sampling is usually undertaken between 9 and 11 weeks of pregnancy by transcervical methods and up to 13 weeks by the transabdominal method, with about 10 weeks being optimum for both. You will be asked to lie flat on a table and the lights will be dimmed while an ultrasound examination of your baby is made. This is important in establishing just where the baby is, where the placenta is and also the exact stage of pregnancy. The ultrasound machine will be kept on during the procedure. (See page 87 about ultrasound tests.)

What happens next depends on whether it's transabdominal or transcervical CVS. Sometimes the position of the placenta may be the determining factor because if it's stuck to the front of the womb transabdominal CVS is easier, whereas if it's stuck to the back transcervical may be easier. Sometimes a particular centre prefers to do it one way rather than the other, simply because that's the technique they are best at. Since experience is a great determinant in risk factors arising from this procedure, you should feel secure with whichever method a particular hospital practises.

Of the two methods, transabdominal appears to be safer (although results of trials are still awaited) because there is no need to go through the cervix, with its attendant potential for introducing infection. However, there appears to be little or no difference in spontaneous miscarriage rates between the two methods.

Before transcervical CVS your cervix may be swabbed to check that there is no infection present. You will need to have a full bladder. You will be asked to lift up your legs, which will then be held apart in stirrups at the foot of the bed. This might be deeply inelegant, but unless we are contortionists, very few of us can manage to hold our legs in that position for more than a minute or so. A metal speculum will be inserted into your vagina, to hold the walls apart and give a clear view of your cervix. The speculum usually feels very cold. A catheter (a thin hollow tube made either of bendy stainless steel or of disposable plastic) will be inserted through the vagina, then through the cervix and pushed towards the chorionic villi under the direction of ultrasound. A small amount of villi are then aspirated using suction. Although it sounds quite unpleasant to have a suction tube pushed through your cervix, most women do not find that it hurts, especially if they are able to relax during the procedure.

After the procedure, the baby will be checked again on ultrasound and you will be asked to lie still for a bit. There may be some slight bleeding, which is just from blood vessels in the vagina which have been knocked during the procedure.

This type of CVS will not be offered if you have any sort of untreated vaginal infection (because of the risks of introducing this infection into the amniotic fluid), or if you come for CVS after 12 weeks. If you have a fibroid low in the uterus, which might impede the passage of the catheter, abdominal CVS would be preferable.

If you are having transabdominal CVS, you will find it very similar to an amniocentesis. Using ultrasound as a guide, a thin hollow needle, similar in size and appearance to the one used for amnios, will be inserted through the skin of the abdomen and womb in order to reach the edge of the placenta. A small sample of chorionic villi will then be withdrawn by suction.

If you have a rhesus negative blood group, you may be given an anti-D injection following the procedure. However, many centres feel that this may not be worthwhile. Although there is a theoretical possibility of the baby's blood escaping into your circulation, given that 0.1 ml of fetal blood is required for sensitization and that this represents half the total blood volume of a nine-week-old fetus, it is unlikely in practice.

Practicalities Wear separates, so that you do not have to undress completely. Take a spare pair of knickers in case they get covered in ultrasound gel. Although you are usually asked to have a full bladder for an ultrasound examination in early pregnancy, abdominal CVS requires an empty bladder. Transcervical CVS requires a full bladder.

After both types of procedure, you will be asked to rest a while before leaving. Once again, it would be preferable to have your partner with you. The general recommendations about rest following the procedure that were outlined for amniocentesis should be followed – you don't have to rest, but you'll probably feel a lot more secure emotionally and physically if you do. Following the procedure you should be on the alert for any sign of infection, such as a raised temperature or, if you've had transabdominal CVS, any leakage of amniotic fluid. If you have had transcervical CVS you should ask for advice about when you should resume lovemaking. You may have a little vaginal bleeding or staining that is blood-tinged in the days following this type of CVS, and this is to be expected because the catheter has probably damaged the delicate vaginal walls. Don't use a tampon to prevent the bleeding if this is the case.

Risks

With transcervical CVS there is a risk of infection which can be life-threatening to the mother unless it is treated quickly with appropriate antibiotics. There is about the same small risk of infection following transabdominal CVS as there is from amniocentesis. In the grand scheme of things infection is a minor consideration, in comparison to the three major concerns about CVS – the rate of spontaneous miscarriage following the procedure, possible damage to the baby and worries about ambiguous test results.

Miscarriage rate   Fortuitously, as this book was being written, the results of the Medical Research Council European Trial of chorionic villus sampling were published in the *Lancet*. This study followed hard on the heels of another large trial of CVS carried out in Canada. What both studies wanted to establish was the risk of miscarriage from CVS and whether it was safer than second trimester amniocentesis in this regard.

One of the difficulties that has beset a proper assessment of the risk of spontaneous miscarriage following CVS has been that the procedure is carried out at a time of pregnancy when miscarriage is at its most common, that is, before 12 weeks.

Although the European results revealed that a woman allocated to CVS had a 4.6 per cent less chance of a successful pregnancy outcome than a woman allocated to second trimester amniocentesis, these figures don't tell the whole story. For instance, terminations following a diagnosis of chromosome abnormality might have removed cases that would have miscarried spontaneously at a later stage of pregnancy. The Canadian trial showed a much less marked difference between the two procedures. The consensus of opinion seems to be that amniocentesis, with a loss rate of probably 0.5 to 1 in every 100 in the best hands, compares favourably with CVS which has a loss rate, in the best hands, of between 2 and 3 in every 100 procedures. There is no doubt that skill of the operator is a very considerable influence on the figures and it may have biased the MRC trial since not all centres involved had the same level of expertise. Some centres, for instance, would claim that their loss rate from CVS was only 1 in 100. Because of this, you should certainly insist on having CVS undertaken in a large centre with an extensive experience of the technique. A suitable level of expertise would involve the operator in at least 50 procedures of this type a year.

Once again, the question you most want answered is, 'If miscarriage is going to happen after CVS, when will it take place?' – in other words, 'When can I consider myself free of the risk of miscarriage?' Unfortunately, as with amniocentesis, there isn't a simple answer. Miscarriage is an ever-present threat, particularly in early pregnancy, and although one would like to say, 'Well, if miscarriage hasn't happened within a week, you're OK', one can't be as certain as this.

Possible damage to the baby There has been a question mark over the use of CVS recently following a report from a centre in Oxford of four babies with limb or combined limb and facial abnormalities, all of whose mothers had had CVS in early pregnancy. This prompted subsequent reports of limb defects, some combined with facial abnormalities, following CVS from a number of countries, including Italy where CVS is a very popular procedure. In general, however, the studies were reassuring. Such abnormalities are really very rare indeed, although the possibility that it was CVS that caused these defects has not been discounted. It might be that such defects are associated with very early CVS and following these reports, CVS is now very rarely carried out before nine weeks.

Concerns over accuracy Because of the way in which CVS is undertaken, contamination of the specimen by maternal cells is much more likely than in amniocentesis. Considerable efforts are made to avoid this and these days maternal contamination is not the problem it once was. Evidently, if the baby is a girl, it is more difficult to assess whether it is the baby's cells or the mother's that are being cultured, but be assured that laboratories are very alert and this is a rare problem.

Because the cells in the chorionic villi are living cells, it is possible to look at direct preparations of cells. However, because of concerns about the accuracy of what is being seen, these cells have to be cultured as well, just to make sure. We saw in the section on amniocentesis that when some cells in cell cultures replicate, they alter in a subtle way from the original cells. Some of this alteration, which results in false abnormalities, may be due to culture conditions and is called pseudomosaicism. In CVS true mosaicism occurs – that is a condition in which different cell types are found within the same cell culture, even though, theoretically, they should all be the same. The reason behind this is that the placenta (and remember that the villi are of the same material as the placenta) does sometimes have a slightly different cellular type from the baby. It is thought that altered cell type in the placenta may account for some otherwise unexplained cases of poor fetal growth, although the baby of course is chromosomally normal. It may also be a cause of early miscarriage. The obvious problem here is that if there is an abnormality in the cell culture, one can't be sure whether it's one that's present in the baby. Again it's a problem that cytogenetics laboratories are very aware of, which is why CVS samples take far more time to process than samples obtained by amniocenteses. Some mixtures of cells seen after CVS are so rare in liveborn babies that further testing is undertaken which may show that the initial result was false. About 2 per cent of CVS results are ambiguous and another 1 per cent of samples will fail to culture at all. In both these situations, a further sample will need to be obtained using amniocentesis or cordocentesis.

Getting the results

Laboratories differ in the way that they process CVS specimens, but in general results are available within 10–20 days and usually by 12–13 weeks of pregnancy. As with amniocentesis, a 'normal' CVS result means that there are the normal number of chromosomes and that they are of the normal shape and size. The baby's sex can be accurately determined. No information about specific single gene defects will have been obtained, unless this was the reason for the CVS in the first place. No information about the presence or absence of physical abnormality will have been obtained.

Overview

The main advantage of CVS is that of early diagnosis, which should ensure a result six or seven weeks before that obtained with conventionally timed amniocentesis. This may be very important to you. However, CVS is undoubtedly a higher risk procedure than amniocentesis, not just because of procedure-related miscarriage, which in the best hands may not be significantly more likely than after amniocentesis, but because of subsequent doubts about the results of the test. If early results are all important, this is the procedure for you. If not, then this procedure is most appropriate for those with a specific reason for having prenatal diagnosis (such as history of handicap). If you are having antenatal testing for reasons of maternal age alone, are happy to wait for your results and do not want invasive testing, then triple test and ultrasound may be more appropriate for you. If you are an older woam and you want specific diagnosis, as opposed to screening, opt for amniocentesis rather than CVS.

8   Fetal blood sampling – cordocentesis

Fetal blood sampling is the last of the three surgical techniques for obtaining fetal material for testing. In this technique a hollow needle is passed through the mother's abdomen and womb and into the umbilical vein. This blood vessel is located in the baby's umbilical cord which also contains other blood vessels (the umbilical arteries). This type of fetal blood sampling is called cordocentesis but there are two other types: hepatocentesis, where a blood sample is taken from the baby's liver, and cardiocentesis, where a blood sample is taken directly from the baby's heart.

Because of the very special skills required to undertake this procedure safely, fetal blood sampling is only available in the largest teaching hospitals and you may therefore have to travel some distance for it. Although it can be used to obtain the same information as amniocentesis, fetal blood sampling has a wider application, including detection of fetal infection, assessment of your baby's state of health in late pregnancy and diagnosis and treatment of blood disorders.

Background   As you will see in the section on biochemical screening (page 129), the blood systems of mother and baby never actually mix during pregnancy. So, if you take a sample directly from the baby's blood system – and the umbilical vein is the most accessible vessel containing the baby's blood – this blood will reflect the baby's health in the same way that a blood sample taken from us would reflect our health. In addition white blood cells contain the same complement of genetic material as all other cells and can therefore be used, in just the same way as the cells obtained through amnios or

CVS, for karyotyping. The one important advantage, however, of using blood cells for this purpose is that they are living cells and require no culture, so karyotyping can be done very rapidly – sometimes within 48 hours. This speedy diagnosis is essential in some situations. For instance, where a physical malformation has been discovered in the baby during an ultrasound scan, rapid karyotyping following cordocentesis may reveal either that the baby is chromosomally normal or that it has a much more extensive handicap than was revealed by the scan. Such information is of vital importance to the parents in decision-making.

Rapid karyotyping is only one benefit of fetal blood sampling. It is also used for a variety of other conditions which we consider later in the chapter.

How and when fetal blood sampling is undertaken

Because your baby's blood vessels are so tiny and so fragile, fetal blood sampling is not possible before 18 weeks of pregnancy. It can be carried out at any time of pregnancy thereafter.

Just as with amniocentesis, you will be asked to lie flat on a table. The obstetrician will first take a detailed look at your baby with ultrasound and will then keep the ultrasound machine on throughout the procedure (see page 87). A hollow needle is used, longer and slightly thicker than for amniocentesis. Under ultrasound control, the needle will be pushed through the mother's abdomen and womb and into the umbilical vein, close to its connection with the placenta. A tiny amount of sterile salty water is then injected into the blood vessel. From the turbulence seen on the ultrasound screen, the obstetrician can be sure that he has inserted the needle in the umbilical vein, rather than the umbilical artery.

About 1–4 ml of blood (a really tiny amount) is withdrawn, depending on the age of the baby and the reason for the fetal blood sampling.

You will be asked to lie still for a bit after the blood is withdrawn and your baby will be closely observed on ultrasound.

Practicalities   Wear separates rather than a dress or dungarees and take a spare pair of knickers in case the pair you're wearing get covered with the ultrasound gel.

Before you have fetal blood sampling, make a list of all the queries you have both about the technique and what the results might mean. Sit down with your partner and your obstetrician and discuss them all. You will find that the types of doctor who undertake fetal blood sampling are people of infinite patience and kindness who not only are technically excellent but who also really understand what the couples coming to them are going through.

If you are pregnant and having fetal blood sampling, the chances are that either you already know that your baby is at risk or you have already been through the testing mill. Perhaps you have had an abnormal biochemical screen or an ultrasound scan that wasn't as reassuring as it should be and further testing has been suggested. Perhaps you have recently been diagnosed as having an infection such as toxoplasmosis. Waiting to have fetal blood sampling, never mind waiting for the results, is as stressful an experience as you're ever likely to go through. You will need every bit of emotional support available during the actual procedure. Try to ensure that your partner is with you, or another close friend. If possible, get someone else to drive you both home afterwards. Try to ensure, by making arrangements in advance if necessary, that you both have time to yourselves when you get back home. Give yourself an easy week following fetal blood sampling.

As with amniocentesis, you should be on the look-out for

leaking amniotic fluid or any rise in your temperature. Ask the obstetrician if there are any special precautions that you should take and when results are likely to be available. Following fetal blood sampling, it's most likely that the obstetrician will contact you directly.

Risks

The maternal complication rate is very small, although one case of amnionitis (infection in the amniotic fluid) has been reported. Risk of spontaneous miscarriage following the procedure is dependent on both the skill of the doctor undertaking it and also the reason for fetal blood sampling. For instance, if your baby is thought to have a chromosomal abnormality, and does indeed have one, miscarriage might have occurred whether or not you had fetal blood sampling. If miscarriage is going to happen – as it does following between 1 and 2 in every 100 procedures – it usually occurs within a week of the sampling.

As with amniocentesis, if no blood can be sampled after two needle insertions, the attempt should be abandoned. The same considerations about blood typing (if you have rhesus negative blood) apply.

Indications for fetal blood sampling

Prenatal diagnosis of blood disorders When fetal blood sampling was first introduced it was used in the main for the diagnosis of blood disorders such as haemophilia, thalassaemia, etc. However, since then new DNA technology has meant that a sample of the baby's blood is no longer required and that first trimester testing (principally using CVS) is now possible. But there are still women who will have fetal blood sampling for this reason because they have been referred too late in pregnancy to have CVS, or for those conditions where linkage studies are necessary and there are no key relatives alive.

Prenatal diagnosis of metabolic disorders There are almost 100 inherited metabolic conditions (see Introduction and Chapter 9 for further details) for which accurate biochemical diagnosis is available. Diagnosis from fetal blood samples can be made within a few hours and this speed of analysis may be important, particularly if late referral has meant that the mother's pregnancy is well advanced.

Prenatal diagnosis of infection If a woman catches an infection such as German measles (rubella virus) in pregnancy, there may be severe consequences for the baby depending on gestation at the time of infection. However, just because the mother has an infection doesn't mean that the baby will have it as well. For instance, 1 in 10 babies whose mothers catch rubella in the first three months of pregnancy will not be infected or affected by the virus. Later in pregnancy, only 50 per cent of babies will be infected and only 25 per cent affected by the rubella virus. A blood sample taken after 22 weeks (when the baby's immune system is properly developed) can determine whether the baby has been infected but not necessarily whether it has been affected unless there are physical signs of damage which will show up on an ultrasound scan. Take, for example, cytomegalovirus, the most common cause of mental handicap in Britain. About 5 per cent of infected babies will develop major neurological problems but unfortunately there is no magic wand that can tell parents whether their baby is one of the 95 per cent or one of the 5 per cent. Similarly with toxoplasmosis infection, only 10 per cent of babies infected in the first trimester of pregnancy (and that's only 10 per cent of the 15 per cent of babies who will contract the infection from their mothers – meaning that 85 per cent of babies will neither be infected nor affected) will develop congenital toxoplasmosis. This type of testing is wonderful if it reveals definitively that your baby does not have an infection but you should be aware that the reverse side of the coin does not necessarily provide you with a clear–cut decision path and you may end up even more anxious than you were before. Two other infective agents, parvovirus B19 and chickenpox (Varicella Zoster virus) are also the subject of this sort of testing.

Assessment of small for dates babies Sometimes babies in the womb are smaller than average, but they are nevertheless healthy. Sometimes they are small because they are sick. Taking a sample of the baby's blood can reveal the true state of the baby's health and can be a crucial guide in determining when and how to deliver the baby. Acid base status is a way of determining how acidic the baby's blood is, and thus whether the baby is getting enough oxygen (oxygen is needed to keep the baby's blood at the correct chemical balance). A number of other chemicals can be measured too, which will give a broader picture of the state of the baby's health. These investigations would only be carried out, however, in pregnancies that are known to be at high risk.

Karyotyping

We have already seen that fetal blood sampling can be important in establishing a karyotype following detection of fetal malformation at ultrasound. If very extensive malformation has been discovered and a couple have opted for termination, it is paradoxically all the more important to have fetal blood sampling in order to establish the baby's genotype. If there is a genetic abnormality in addition to the physical malformation, it will be of crucial importance in counselling for the future.

Other reasons for wanting a speedy karyotype are when cell

culture from earlier amniocentesis has failed, or when previous cell culture has provided an ambiguous result (mosaicism or pseudomosaicism). A high risk indication following biochemical screening may also be a reason for wanting rapid karyotyping, rather than waiting three or five weeks for the results of an amniocentesis.

Diagnosis of Fragile X-linked mental retardation   Fragile X syndrome, occurring in 1 per 1,000 live male births, is second only to Down's syndrome as a genetic cause of mental retardation. Demonstration of the Fragile X chromosome is easiest in fetal white blood cells, hence the preferred use of cordocentesis rather than CVS or amniocentesis to obtain material for diagnosis of this condition.

Overview

Fetal blood sampling is an option only if there is a specific reason for rapid karyotyping or for fetal diagnosis. It can only be carried out after 18 weeks of pregnancy but set against the disadvantage of the lateness of the procedure is the speed with which results can be obtained, something which may be of particular importance. It is only available in specialist hospitals. ·

9   **Biochemical Screening**

Taking a sample of a pregnant woman's blood in order to find out more about the health of her baby sounds like a good idea. It is simple, doesn't hurt and carries no risks for either mother or baby. So why can't women just have a blood test during pregnancy and do away with things like amniocentesis?

To understand why this is not possible but why testing the mother's blood can give you important information about the baby, you need to know something about the blood systems of both mother and developing baby.

The placenta is anchored in the wall of the womb by little frond-like growths called villi (from the Latin for finger). The villi, which the baby supplies with lots of blood via its umbilical cord, dangle, rather like fronds of seaweed in a rock pool, in little lakes of the mother's blood, deep in the wall of the womb. Some substances can escape from the baby's blood through the thin skin of the villi and thence into the lakes of the mother's blood – gases such as oxygen and carbon dioxide and little molecules such as hormones. But the baby's blood is firmly enclosed in each little frond by an overlying layer of 'skin', just like the inside of the seaweed is enclosed by its outer covering. This ensures that the mother's and baby's blood supplies never actually mix. But sometimes the overlying 'skin' of the villi tears, allowing a small amount of the baby's blood or some of the 'skin cells' (actually known as trophoblast cells) to escape into the mother's blood supply. The mother's blood will then contain substances produced by the baby and a few – a very few – of the baby's blood cells.

If you could isolate the baby's blood cells from the mother's blood, you could of course use these cells for direct testing and chromosome analysis in the same way that you can use cells obtained by amniocentesis or CVS. But because there are so few cells – it is estimated that there is just one of the baby's cells to every thousand million of the mother's blood cells – it's a bit like looking for a needle in a haystack. All attempts to find a simple and cheap way of isolating these few cells from a sample of the mother's blood have come to nothing. However, some recent advances look more promising. Fetal red blood cells differ from most adult red blood cells in that they have a nucleus (the central portion of a cell that contains the chromosomes). Using a novel process involving magnets, the sample can be selectively 'cleansed' of maternal cells – first the red blood cells without nuclei, then white blood cells – leaving a final mix of both fetal and maternal nucleated red blood cells. In this mixture, there is about one fetal red blood cell to every 10,000 maternal red blood cells. Because fetal haemoglobin (the pigment that makes blood appear red) is not the same as adult haemoglobin, the fetal cells can then be picked out using a high density optical system. This process has the potential to be both swift and cheap and is currently under review. There is no doubt that in the next five years, maternal blood testing will become a reality.

All maternal blood tests currently in use for screening purposes work on the principle that the mother's blood contains chemicals which have got into her blood from the baby and that the levels of these chemicals may provide an indication as to the health of the baby.

There are two main tests which use a sample of the mother's blood. One, which is very commonly used in British hospitals, screens for spina bifida and other similar handicaps and is called maternal serum alphafetoprotein (MSAFP). The other test, which is becoming more and more common, is not only used to screen for spina bifida but also for Down's syndrome. This second test is known variously as triple test, the Barts test or simply biochemical screening.

The important thing to stress is that these are not tests

where you get a straight yes or no answer to a given question. They are screening tests. A good way to think of these sorts of test is as fishermen's nets trawling for a particular type of fish. At the end of the day, the net may be full. Most of the shoal may have been caught but some will have escaped and, as you might imagine, there are a fair few other hapless fish caught up in the net by mistake. Such is screening.

So before you read any further, just remember that if you screen positive to any of the tests discussed below, it doesn't mean that you have a handicapped baby – but neither, as we have discussed in earlier chapters, does a screen negative result guarantee the health of your baby.

10   MSAFP

Maternal serum alphafetoprotein or MSAFP for short is used to assess how likely it is that a woman will have a baby with one of the family of handicaps known as neural tube defects (NTD). The best known of these handicaps are spina bifida and anencephaly. In spina bifida, the neural tube that should enclose the central nervous cord is incomplete, rather like a pipe with a hole in it. Sometimes skin has grown over the hole (a closed lesion), but much more often it is open. In anencephaly, the covering of the brain is incomplete. This handicap is incompatible with life and anencephalic babies always die at or very shortly after birth. NTDs are much more common in some parts of Britain than others; for instance there is a high incidence in some parts of Scotland, South Wales and East Anglia, whereas they are relatively uncommon in the South East of England. The cause of NTDs is not known but they are thought to be multifactorial in origin, which means basically that a number of different factors, both inherited and environmental, act together to cause them. Interestingly, in women having twins, it is very rare for both twins to have a neural tube defect.

A recent MRC study has shown definitively that taking folic acid supplements before and after conception can help in the prevention of NTDs for those with a previously affected child, reducing incidence by 72 per cent. Whether supplements would reduce the incidence in the whole population is not known, although the government has recently recommended folic acid supplements of 400 mg daily for women in early pregnancy. It is possible that the problem is not that women who have babies with NTDs have low intakes of folates but that they are unable to use the folates that they do take in effectively. Folic acid-rich foods such as fortified breakfast cereals and dark green vegetables should be high on your list of food priorities both before and during pregnancy.

The incidence of NTDs is about 4–5 per 1,000, although this varies quite a bit depending on where you live, from 7–8 per 1,000 in Wales to 1–2 per 1,000 in London. If you've already had a baby with a neural tube defect, the risk of having another is increased tenfold. However, it is important to point out that 95 per cent of babies with NTDs are born to couples with no history of NTD in the family.

The chemical which is the basis of the test is a protein, alphafetoprotein (AFP but also written as αFP) which is made by the baby's liver and then excreted with the baby's urine into the pool of amniotic fluid (see amniocentesis, page 104). There are large quantities of AFP in the skin and muscles of babies and if there is an open hole in the skin, as there is in some NTDs, it leaks out, so that much larger concentrations of AFP are found in the fluid than normal. This makes open lesions much easier to detect than closed lesions. Some of this AFP gets into the mother's blood across the placenta, and the higher the concentration in the fluid, the more that gets across the placenta.

How and when the test is done

This test is done between 16 and 18 weeks of pregnancy in most health regions, simply by taking a small sample of blood. It is very often done after an initial ultrasound scan because by dating the pregnancy from one particular head measurement (the biparietal diameter) the detection rate for open spina bifida lesions is increased from 79 per cent to 91 per cent. In general, MSAFP is about 90 per cent accurate as a screening test. False negatives are rare but false positives are, unfortunately, quite common.

You may find that you live in a region which does not feel

that it is worthwhile doing this test, simply because the incidence is very low in your part of the country. Your region may prefer to put its money into more intensive ultrasound screening for its pregnant women. Some regions have extended the use of this blood sample and now screen for both NTDs and Down's syndrome with triple test.

Screening has resulted in a reduction in birth prevalence of NTDs among screened women of 75 per cent, although it is known that this reduction isn't entirely due to screening – the natural incidence of these handicaps does seem to be falling.

Getting the results

The results of AFP tests should be back within a week or so, but all regions vary. When you have the blood sample taken, ask how long it will be before you get the result and how you will receive it. You may get an 'If you don't hear from us, assume everything's OK' answer. This isn't very satisfactory and can leave you feeling anxious for some time. It may be possible for you to leave a stamped addressed card which can be sent to you on receipt of a negative screen result.

Results will be expressed as a number that gives a risk rate, usually as something called an MoM or Multiple of the Median. This sounds complicated but it's really just a way of expressing your risk relative to others. This MoM number can be adjusted according to your weight, race, age and week of pregnancy.

If you have a low AFP level, you will not normally be retested. This is partly because levels go up anyway as pregnancy progresses. A repeat test for a high level will either produce a result within normal limits if your dates were incorrect, or continue to be high.

Problems

Nine out of ten women who have a raised level of AFP do not have a handicapped baby. The problem with AFP testing is that it is not very specific. As you can see from the figure above, there is quite an overlap between normal babies and babies with an NTD. It is also a test which is very dependent on you having got your dates right, which is why a prior ultrasound scan can be important. Let me explain: AFP levels rise at a consistent rate during the first two-thirds of pregnancy. If you think you are 16 weeks, but are in fact 18 weeks pregnant, you will appear to have an abnormally high level of AFP for your dates, although it might be quite normal for 18 weeks.

What if you have a high level of AFP? As we have seen, having a high level of AFP doesn't mean that you have a handicapped baby. The test may be repeated and if the level is still high for your stage of pregnancy, you will be offered an amniocentesis. Although high AFP levels are found in quite a number of normal pregnancies, the difference between normal and abnormal pregnancies is much more marked in amniotic fluid levels of AFP. The amnios for AFP determination are carried out in just the same way as the amnios described on page 104, although there is of course no need for cell culture because it's the actual fluid, not the cells it contains, that is important.

Alternatively, you might simply be offered a further, more detailed scan, sometimes in another hospital which has a higher level of scanning expertise. You might think that neural tube defects ought to be spotted by ultrasound alone. Anencephaly is almost always picked up with ultrasound but it can be missed, as can many of the smaller lesions associated with spina bifida. Read the section on ultrasound for further information.

There are one or two other specific instances where high AFP levels have a demonstrable cause other than NTDs.

Previous bleeding in pregnancy, for instance, is a relatively common cause of high AFP levels. Kidney and gut problems in the baby are also a possibility, although a very unlikely one. There are also some rare instances where the combination of a high AFP level with other factors, such as a very small amount of amniotic fluid or the signs of possible miscarriage, sounds clear alarm bells as to the health of the baby.

But one of the best of all reasons for higher than usual levels of AFP is that you have more than one baby. Curiously, higher levels of AFP are associated with identical rather than non-identical twins. A further curiosity is that consistently higher levels of AFP are associated with boys than girls. AFP levels are also closely linked to the mother's weight and race, with thin women having consistently higher AFP levels than fat women. Such findings may go some way towards explaining why elevated levels are so often found to be without cause.

In fact you should be aware that at birth no reason at all can be found for elevated AFP levels in 50 per cent of babies whose mothers' blood contained high levels of AFP in pregnancy. Does this mean that, if no cause can be found for an elevated AFP, you should ignore the result? Evidence suggests that the finding should be viewed in rather the same way as you view a hazard road sign, like the one with the leaping deer on it. It doesn't mean that a deer is waiting to jump in front of your car around the next corner – it just means that you should be aware of the possibility. In the same way, unexplained high AFP levels are sometimes indicators of possible hazards ahead. For instance it is strongly suspected that problems with the placenta are responsible for some unexplained high AFP levels. Many obstetricians would therefore think it a prudent precaution to monitor your pregnancy and particularly the baby's growth following such a finding.

What if you have an unexpectedly low MSAFP finding? While there is an association with Down's syndrome as you will see later, the prevailing evidence suggests that women

with low MSAFP levels do not face the same possible risks of
adverse pregnancy outcome, such as poor growth of the baby,
as those associated with unexplained elevated levels.

Overview

MSAFP is a test which may require nerves of steel because
there is usually a three-week gap between having a positive
screen result and having a subsequent scan, repeat test and/or
amniocentesis – and your baby may have been normal all
along. Of all the tests outlined in this book, this, together
with triple test, is the one that seems simplest at the outset but
which you may end up wishing you had never embarked
upon. If you are going to opt for AFP testing, you might
prefer to have the triple test, which has the advantage of also
picking up Down's syndrome.

11   Triple Test

Triple test is really an extension of MSAFP in that, in addition to measuring AFP for NTD screening, two other chemicals (two hormones called unconjugated oestriol and human chorionic gonadotrophin) are measured. The levels of these two chemicals, together with a woman's age, are used to give an estimate of risk for Down's syndrome.

This test goes by a variety of names, which can make things a bit confusing. You may hear this test just called biochemical testing, or the triple test (because three different substances are measured), or the Barts test (because St Bartholomew's Hospital was where it was first used). You may also hear it simply called maternal serum screening.

The table in Figure 7 can be used to calculate the odds of a woman's risk of having a Down's baby at a particular age. You should view these risk figures rather as, for instance, you would view the odds quoted for a woman being killed as she crosses the road. In other words, they are composite figures which do not reflect individual circumstances, merely an overall risk. To calculate individual risk for road crossing effectively, you would need more information, such as the speed of traffic. Also are we talking about an old lady attempting to cross the M25 or about a 19-year-old crossing a quiet cul-de-sac? Triple test is a way of arriving at an individual estimate of risk of having a Down's baby, using additional pieces of information unique to you. Risk quotes can be altered quite dramatically from, say, 1 in 126 for a woman who is 40 on her delivery date, to 1 in 6,000 following triple test. Over 70 per cent of all 40-year-old women can be shown, following triple test, to have an individual risk LESS than that

Years	Completed months											
---	0	1	2	3	4	5	6	7	8	9	10	11
25	1:1376	1:1372	1:1367	1:1363	1:1358	1:1353	1:1348	1:1343	1:1338	1:1333	1:1328	1:1322
26	1:1317	1:1311	1:1306	1:1300	1:1294	1:1289	1:1283	1:1277	1:1271	1:1264	1:1258	1:1252
27	1:1245	1:1239	1:1232	1:1225	1:1219	1:1212	1:1205	1:1198	1:1191	1:1183	1:1176	1:1169
28	1:1161	1:1154	1:1146	1:1138	1:1130	1:1123	1:1115	1:1107	1:1099	1:1090	1:1082	1:1074
29	1:1065	1:1057	1:1048	1:1040	1:1031	1:1022	1:1014	1:1005	1: 996	1: 987	1: 978	1: 969
30	1: 960	1: 951	1: 942	1: 932	1: 923	1: 914	1: 905	1: 895	1: 886	1: 877	1: 867	1: 858
31	1: 848	1: 839	1: 829	1: 820	1: 810	1: 801	1: 791	1: 782	1: 772	1: 763	1: 753	1: 744
32	1: 734	1: 725	1: 716	1: 706	1: 697	1: 687	1: 678	1: 669	1: 660	1: 650	1: 641	1: 632
33	1: 623	1: 614	1: 605	1: 596	1: 587	1: 578	1: 570	1: 561	1: 552	1: 544	1: 535	1: 527
34	1: 518	1: 510	1: 502	1: 494	1: 486	1: 478	1: 470	1: 462	1: 454	1: 446	1: 439	1: 431
35	1: 424	1: 416	1: 409	1: 402	1: 395	1: 387	1: 381	1: 374	1: 367	1: 360	1: 354	1: 347
36	1: 341	1: 334	1: 328	1: 322	1: 316	1: 310	1: 304	1: 298	1: 292	1: 287	1: 281	1: 275
37	1: 270	1: 265	1: 259	1: 254	1: 249	1: 244	1: 239	1: 235	1: 230	1: 225	1: 221	1: 216
38	1: 212	1: 207	1: 203	1: 199	1: 195	1: 191	1: 187	1: 183	1: 179	1: 175	1: 171	1: 168
39	1: 164	1: 161	1: 157	1: 154	1: 151	1: 147	1: 144	1: 141	1: 138	1: 135	1: 132	1: 129
40	1: 126	1: 124	1: 121	1: 118	1: 116	1: 113	1: 111	1: 108	1: 106	1: 103	1: 101	1: 99
41	1: 97	1: 94	1: 92	1: 90	1: 88	1: 86	1: 84	1: 82	1: 81	1: 79	1: 77	1: 75
42	1: 73	1: 72	1: 70	1: 69	1: 67	1: 65	1: 64	1: 63	1: 61	1: 60	1: 58	1: 57
43	1: 56	1: 54	1: 53	1: 52	1: 51	1: 49	1: 48	1: 47	1: 46	1: 45	1: 44	1: 43
44	1: 42	1: 41	1: 40	1: 39	1: 38	1: 37	1: 36	1: 35	1: 35	1: 34	1: 33	1: 32
45	1: 31	1: 31	1: 30	1: 29	1: 29	1: 28	1: 27	1: 27	1: 26	1: 25	1: 25	1: 24
46	1: 24	1: 23	1: 22	1: 22	1: 21	1: 21	1: 20	1: 20	1: 19	1: 19	1: 18	1: 18
47	1: 17	1: 17	1: 17	1: 16	1: 16	1: 15	1: 15	1: 15	1: 14	1: 14	1: 14	1: 13
48	1: 13	1: 13	1: 12	1: 12	1: 12	1: 11	1: 11	1: 11	1: 11	1: 10	1: 10	1: 10
49	1:9.5	1:9.2	1:9.0	1:8.8	1:8.5	1:8.3	1:8.1	1:7.9	1:7.7	1:7.5	1:7.3	1:7.1

Figure 7 Risk of a Down's syndrome term pregnancy according to maternal age, in years and months, at the expected date of delivery. (*From* Antenatal and Neonatal Screening, *Ed. N. Wald, Oxford University Press, 1984*)

normally quoted for a 35-year-old (the usual amnio cut-off age).

For some reason, as yet to be adequately explained, blood levels of AFP are lower in women carrying a baby affected by Down's syndrome. However, a low AFP result in itself is not sufficiently accurate as a screening test and were it to be used alone there would be a very large number of false positives. Low levels of maternal blood oestriol and high levels of maternal HCG (human chorionic gonadotrophin) are both associated with Down's, but once again, the level of each in itself is insufficient to use as a screening test. But measurement of all three markers together with the mother's age and gestation is far more predictive, allowing 60 per cent of all Down's babies to be detected.

Just like the AFP test, this is not a yes or no type of test. It's a screening test. All it will tell you is whether you have an increased risk of having a baby with either a neural tube defect or Down's syndrome. If you are shown to be at increased risk, you can then opt for further diagnostic testing, such as amniocentesis. An important point to note is that a screen negative result is not a guarantee that your baby does not have Down's as this test can only detect two out of every three Down's babies.

You need to think carefully about this test before you have it. It carries no risk to yourself or your baby but if you do have a positive screen result, you may go through a lot of anxiety and worry and still have a healthy baby at the end of it all. As with the AFP test, you need to know that a positive result does not mean you are carrying a handicapped baby – it simply means that there is a greater risk of having a baby with a handicap, in the same way that you have a greater risk as you get older. And although you know that older women are at greater risk, I'm quite sure that the vast majority of your friends who have had later pregnancies have had healthy babies.

At the moment, only older women are offered specific testing for Down's syndrome, even though 65 per cent of Down's babies are born to women under 35. But younger women couldn't all be given amnios because many more normal babies would be miscarried because of the amnio procedure than babies with Down's would be detected. This test might be specially important for older women who may prefer not to have an amniocentesis because of the risk of miscarriage if their risk estimate is low. The importance of this screening test is that for the first time younger women can be screened with a no risk procedure for Down's syndrome.

How and when the test is done

A small amount of blood is taken from the mother between 16 weeks and 23 weeks of pregnancy. The test results may need different interpretation if you have a twin pregnancy or insulin-dependent diabetes. If this is the case, you will need further advice from your gynaecologist before having this test. If you have already had an attempted amniocentesis in this pregnancy, the test cannot be interpreted properly. Like AFP testing, it is important that exact gestation is known before testing.

Getting the results

The result of the screening is reported as either 'screen positive' or 'screen negative', usually within ten days of the test. For this test, a result is provided for all women, even if they screen negative, so at least you don't have to worry about the results being lost.

The cut-off level between screen positive and screen negative is 1 in 250, roughly the risk of a woman of 37 years of age having a Down's baby. You would screen positive, then, if your risk was estimated as being greater than 1 in 250. For those who are as mathematically inept as I am, by the way, a greater risk than 1 in 250 is shown as a smaller number, e.g. 1 in 50, or 1 in 100. A lower risk than 1 in 250 is shown as a bigger number, 1 in 500 or 1 in 1,000. Risk needs to be put in perspective. It may seem to you that 1 in 100 is quite a high risk, but remember that this means that 99 babies are likely to be born without handicap. Nobody can tell you at which level of risk you ought to opt for further testing – older women are often prepared to accept much higher risks than younger women.

If the level of AFP was high, further ultrasound scans or an amniocentesis might be indicated as discussed above in the section on MSAFP testing. If the levels of the other chemicals were abnormal and there was concern about Down's, amniocentesis might be offered. Sometimes another ultrasound scan is all that is required because a further scan may establish that the pregnancy is not as far as, or further on than you thought, thereby causing the results of the test to be reinterpreted and putting you in the screen negative group.

More than 9 out of 10 women will have a screen negative result, where the risk is less than 1 in 250.

What a screen negative result does not do is guarantee that your baby will not have Down's or spina bifida. There is still a chance, although it is only a very small one. This is because the test can detect only two out of every three Down's babies. Almost all cases of anencephaly should be detected and four out of every five of open spina bifida lesions.

Many hospitals now offer this type of screening. It is also available privately at a cost of between £50 and £80. However, if you do have it done privately, remember that you need to have had a dating scan first. Also remember to ask who you will be able to talk to about interpreting the result before having the test.

Triple Test Plus

Decisions made by health authorities as to which screening tests should be offered routinely to women in their area have, of necessity, to be influenced by financial considerations. For instance, there is a test which, when added to triple test, increases the detection rate of Down's syndrome dramatically to between 80 and 90 per cent. It involves measuring the levels of an enzyme, alkaline phosphatase, in a certain type of white blood cell called a neutrophil in a pregnant woman's blood. This is the NAP test. Neutrophils of women carrying Down's babies have more alkaline phosphatase in them than women with normal babies and these particular blood cells therefore take up more of a special type of dye. In practice this means that a laboratory technician has to assess the numbers of neutrophils which contain a deeper colour of dye. Assessing the degree of colour shading is an art in itself, which calls for constant quality control monitoring. All of this means that the test is too costly to be carried out on a nationwide basis, although theoretically it might be introduced if a way could be found to automate it. Triple test plus is currently available from the University of Leeds Down's Syndrome Screening Service (0532 344013, St James's University Hospital, Leeds LS9 7TF) who will send, on request, a sample phial for your blood and some glass slides, together with an explanatory note (for the person taking your blood sample), and a leaflet for you which will give you further details of their triple test plus service. This service costs £88 at the time of writing.

Overview

Triple test has its limitations and it could cause you a great deal of worry. You need to be clear in your own mind what screen positive and screen negative mean *before* you have the test. However, combined with ultrasound scanning, it would appear to offer the best pregnancy screening so far available for all pregnant women. It is particularly valuable to older women who may want an accurate assessment of risk before having an amniocentesis, or for those women who have had a history of miscarriage. A drawback is that it cannot be undertaken until relatively late in pregnancy.

Despite its potential, the experience of introducing triple test on a wider basis has not been a happy one. Part of the problem appears to be that prior explanation or counselling is woefully inadequate. As a result many women who are given a 'screen positive' result assume that their baby has got Down's. The only way to relieve their anxiety – or confirm that their baby has got Down's – is to undertake karyotyping. It is intolerable for these women to be expected to wait for the results of amniocentesis. As a result, the workload of tertiary referral centres has increased dramatically as they are besieged by women with 'screen positive' triple test results, wanting either cordocentesis or detailed ultrasound scanning which would give them a clearer (although not definitive) indication of whether their baby has Down's.

Unfortunately medicine is littered with examples of 'this seems like a good idea' practices, which have been insufficiently thought through. A classic in the field of antenatal diagnosis was the screening programme to detect sickle-cell carriers in the United States. Carrier screening was offered (and even legally enforced in some states). However, there was unsufficient explanation that those with sickle-cell trait (i.e. carriers of sickle-cell disease) were perfectly healthy, with no symptoms of sickle-cell disease at all. As a result, there was discrimination against those with sickle-cell trait by employers and insurance companies. Since those with sickle-cell trait are likely to be black the question of civil rights and racial discrimination was raised and the carrier detection programme was vilified. Triple test screening runs a similar risk of shooting itself in the foot through insufficient prior thought and it may well be, because of the extreme anxieties induced by it and the increased rather than decreased demand for diagnostic antenatal tests caused by it, that triple test will be phased out in favour of ultrasound screening for Down's syndrome, using the nuchal fold indicator (see page 99). Only time will tell.

12   Testing for Toxoplasma

The last type of testing that we shall consider is in many ways very different from those we have already discussed, although many of the issues remain the same. Over the last twenty years there has been a truly dramatic reduction in the number of babies dying either at birth or within a few days of birth. And while twenty, ten and even five years ago, medical effort was largely directed towards the major killers – prematurity and fetal abnormality – less common causes of baby death and handicap are now receiving more attention. One such is infection in pregnancy, particularly the so-called TORCH infections. These are *TO*xoplasma, *R*ubella, *C*ytomegalovirus and *H*erpes.

One of the first things to say about infection in pregnancy is that just because the mother has an infection, it doesn't mean that the baby has to have it too. Nor does it always follow that the more severe the infection in the mother, the more likely the baby is to have it. In fact, thanks to the barrier provided by the placenta, infection in the baby is the exception rather than the rule and is dependent on a number of factors which vary according to the infection. The stage of pregnancy at which the mother caught the infection can be critical. It is also known that transmission rates of infection across the placenta are different in Britain from those found in the United States or France, certainly for toxoplasma and possibly other TORCH infections as well.

Testing for infection poses special problems because although it is relatively easy to establish whether the mother has an infection, it is not so easy to determine the status of the baby. Of even greater concern is the fact that an infected baby may very well not be an affected baby, that is, simply contracting an infection may not result in handicap.

The problems posed by cytomegalovirus (CMV) illustrate the dilemmas very well. It is a common virus and 50 per cent of women will have unknowingly been infected by it by their early twenties. With peak infection rates between the ages of 15 and 35, the possibility of infection in pregnancy is high. Infection at any stage in pregnancy (transmission rates do not vary with stage of pregnancy with CMV) can cause mental handicap and deafness in the baby. These symptoms do not, however, develop until after birth and of approximately 2,000 babies born with a congenital infection (that is, infection acquired in the womb), fewer than 100 will subsequently suffer major handicap. Theoretically it is possible to screen for CMV infections in pregnant women. Theoretically one could then offer cordocentesis (a procedure which carries risk of spontaneous miscarriage, see page 125) to CMV positive women to establish whether the baby was infected, although only a third of these women's babies will prove to be infected. And then what? Offer termination to mothers with infected babies in the knowledge that 95 per cent of them will still, despite the fact that their babies have a CMV infection, have a healthy baby? Were screening of this sort to be adopted, far more healthy babies would die than babies with handicap caused by CMV would be prevented. This is why CMV screening, despite the virus being a major cause of mental handicap, has not been adopted in Britain. It also serves to show the problems that this type of testing for infection would bring in its wake. The long and short of it is that many women would have a quite needless burden of worry and anxiety thrust upon them. Unless there is a very specific reason for taking up CMV testing, please do not think you are being a responsible parent by asking for it. You do not need the incredible anxiety that this test will almost inevitably bring

– just concentrate on the fact that the odds in favour of your baby being unaffected are very heavily stacked.

Toxoplasma is another infection, caused by a microscopic parasite, that poses similar problems to CMV in that current testing is based on detecting the disease rather than detecting handicap. An additional difficulty is that there is very considerable confusion about the implications of Toxoplasma test results, not least among the medical profession. Women can take active steps to avoid infection by Toxoplasma and, crucially, can establish their Toxoplasma status prior to pregnancy. This last is an important point although even this measure may not be ideal since there is a relatively high false positive rate which may falsely reassure. A positive test result prior to pregnancy should not mean that you ignore basic preventive measures.

Like CMV infection, Toxoplasma infection (toxoplasmosis) is a common event, with 30 per cent of 30-year-olds being Toxoplasma positive, rising to 50 per cent of 70-year-olds. Like CMV, infection with Toxoplasma may not be marked by any symptoms, although some people experience ones akin to glandular fever – sore throat, enlarged glands, fatigue, aches and pains, etc. Toxoplasma infection is of importance to two groups of people: immunosuppressed individuals (such as those with AIDS or on immunosuppressive drugs) and pregnant women.

Before going on to the specifics of possible effects in pregnancy, some explanations are needed both about the nature of the beast itself and also of ways to avoid catching it. Toxoplasma gondii is a parasitic organism. Microscopic in size, it comes from a large family of single-celled beasts called Protozoa, the most familiar of which is the amoeba. It can move about only by flexing its body, but its forte is reproduction – it has three different and equally effective ways of reproducing itself by the thousand. The cat, domestic, wild or jungle, is its main host (that is, it requires a cat to complete its

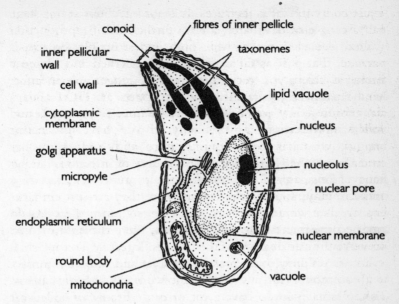

conoid

fibres of inner pellicle

inner pellicular
wall

taxonemes

cell wall

lipid vacuole

cytoplasmic
membrane

nucleus

golgi apparatus

nucleolus

micropyle

nuclear pore

endoplasmic reticulum

nuclear membrane

round body

mitochondria

vacuole

Figure 8a *Toxoplasma gondii* ultrastructure (*Taken from* Introduction to Animal Parasitology *Second Edition, J. D. Smyth, Hodder & Stoughton 1976*)

life cycle) but it also infects many other species of animal including mice, birds, sheep, pigs, goats, cattle, us and, unlikely though it sounds, gondis, a species of North African rodent from which it takes its name.

Knowing the life cycle of this organism is essential because it is the key to preventing infection. When a cat eats a bird or mouse infected by Toxoplasma, the Toxoplasma invades the cells lining the cat's gut. It reproduces itself with abandon until the cat's defence systems cotton on to its presence, and then another form of reproduction takes place in the gut, resulting in a special form of the Toxoplasma which is enclosed in an incredibly tough case or oocyst which is then excreted by the cat in its faeces. It is not infectious at this stage but a couple of days later, after a further bit of reproduction (called sporulation), a well nigh indestructible oocyst is formed. That's it as far as the cat is concerned and it's now immune, thank you very much, and no longer able to infect you. From this you can see that cats' faeces are NOT always dangerous – they are only likely to be infective in the period following infection. This is why, if you have an ancient moggy who has been hunting mice and birds since her kittenhood, she is unlikely to be a source of infection, having long since acquired it, and become immune. Kittens are a more obvious source of infection, since they are just embarking on their hunting careers, but even so, since the cysts do not become infective for 24–48 hours, there is plenty of time to see to the safe disposal of their faeces. Infective Toxoplasmal cysts are unlikely to be present on a cat and ordinary contact with a cat will not put a pregnant woman's unborn baby at risk. Thus if you do have a cat or cats, dispose of soiled cat litter on a daily basis, wearing gloves to do so, and washing your hands afterwards. It is irresponsible to suggest that pregnant women should not touch cats or even keep cats because of the risk of Toxoplasma.

Grass-eating animals acquire Toxoplasma by ingesting soil where cat faeces have been present, the oocysts remaining on the grass and in the earth for many months after the faeces themselves have disappeared. When animals eat the grass, the cysts are ingested, the walls are broken down in the stomach, and the tiny Toxoplasmas inside are released. They invade cells in the body and form little bags or cysts, most notably within muscle tissue, and then multiply within these cysts. Humans can acquire Toxoplasma as a result of poor hygiene after handling soil (when gardening, gloves are advisable and you should always wash your hands afterwards), through not washing food items likely to be contaminated by contact with soil (such as salads and vegetables) and of course, by eating

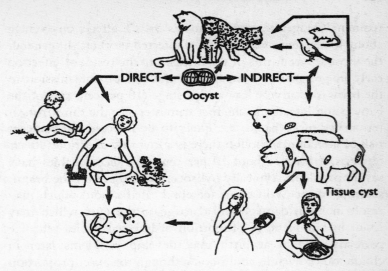

Figure 8b Lifecycle of *toxoplasma gondii* and routes of transmission to humans. (*Taken from* British Medical Journal Vol 305, August 1992, *Dr Susan M. Hall*)

meat from grass-eating animals that is not sufficiently cooked to destroy the tissue cysts.

The penchant of the French for eating undercooked meat results in the majority of French women having already acquired immunity to Toxoplasma by the time they become pregnant. If you have to eat meat raw, use meat that has previously been deep frozen as freezing also kills tissue cysts. You should note that while commercial freezers will reach a low enough temperature ($-20°C$), domestic freezers may not; certainly the freezer compartment of a fridge would not be adequate. The Dutch estimate that in developed countries, meat is the most likely source of Toxoplasma infection. There is also now known to be a risk from drinking unpasteurized goat's milk.

What of the effects of Toxoplasma infection in pregnant

women? Congenital toxoplasmosis or CT affects on average about 40 per cent of the babies of infected mothers. In general, the most severe forms of the disease are the result of infection early in pregnancy, even though the rate of transmission to the baby is relatively low at this stage (10 per cent risk of the baby being infected in the first trimester). In the third trimester, many more babies are likely to be infected (90 per cent risk of infection) although there is a low risk of serious effects obvious at birth. About 10 per cent of infected babies have severe problems, typically hydrocephalus (fluid on the brain), scarring of the brain tissue (cerebral calcification) which may result in brain damage and damage to the eyes which may result in blindness. A proportion of infected babies who are perfectly normal at birth may develop problems later in childhood or even in adulthood although the exact proportion is not known. The problem is usually something called retinochoroiditis (damage to the retina of the eye caused by Toxoplasma cysts) which can cause blindness but more often attacks of reduced vision which usually respond well to drug treatment.

All of this sounds horribly alarming, especially since toxoplasmosis is said to be more common than rubella, but how common is toxoplasmosis in pregnancy? It is thought that about 2 in every 1,000 pregnant women become infected during their pregnancy. It is said that at this infection rate, there are between 500 and 600 cases of congenital infection per annum in the UK, with 10 per cent of them being serious. However, a recent survey conducted by the Public Health Laboratory Service through the British Paediatric Surveillance Unit identified a much smaller number of serious cases than this estimate would suggest (fewer than ten in England and Wales). This means either that the infection rate is not as great as supposed, or that a large number of serious cases are being missed or not followed up long for enough to confirm diagnosis, or that more babies escape unharmed than was previously thought. The British situation is often compared to that in France where a great deal is known about Toxoplasma infection, but as I have already pointed out, infection rates vary from country to country and the French experience cannot therefore be compared directly to that of Britain.

Testing for Toxoplasma in pregnancy involves at least two tests on a sample of a pregnant woman's blood to establish whether she is suffering from toxoplasmosis. These are indirect tests in that they are looking not for Toxoplasma itself, but specific antibodies produced as a consequence of infection by Toxoplasma. Antibodies are the substances made by the body's defence system in response to infection – think of them as the body's infection memory. They are made of special proteins called immunoglobulins which come in four main varieties, each one denoted by an initial. They are written as follows: IgG, IgA, IgE and IgM.

You can think of IgM as being the temporary response to infection by Toxoplasma, rising and then falling soon after infection and IgG as being a lifelong memory of Toxoplasma infection. If there is no evidence of any IgG, then it is generally accepted that the woman has never had toxoplasmosis. If the result is slightly raised then a repeat blood test will be taken at a ten-day interval. If there is a significant increase in the IgG level, it suggests a current infection. A raised IgM would suggest a recent infection. On the face of it this seems fairly straightforward but in reality the situation is rather different. A current infection, in which there are rising levels of IgG over a short time interval, or a situation in which no infection is demonstrated is fairly clear cut, but the middle ground between is very difficult to interpret. For instance, is a 'recent' infection one that was contracted some time before pregnancy even began, or was it contracted during the early stages of pregnancy? This is when knowledge of whether you were immune to Toxoplasma before pregnancy started can be of sanity-preserving importance.

If infection is diagnosed in the mother, the status of the baby needs to be established. Unfortunately this cannot be done before 22 weeks of pregnancy when the baby's immune system is sufficiently developed to allow proper interpretation of antibody testing. A sample of blood is obtained from the baby using cordocentesis. Cordocentesis would be carried out in a teaching hospital. A Toxoplasma Reference Laboratory will be involved and their expertise will help the obstetrician to advise you.

The baby is regarded as infected if there are IgM antibodies in its blood (results take one week) or if innoculation of the sample of blood into mice detects Toxoplasma parasites (results take up to six weeks). If infection was severe enough to cause fetal abnormality, this could be detected with ultrasound scanning. A detailed explanation of cordocentesis and its role in detection of infection is available in Chapter 4.

If the baby is infected but showing no sign of abnormality on scan, a combination of drugs (pyrimethamine and sulphadiazine) may be offered. These are known to be fairly successful in preventing further damage occurring to the baby. If the baby is not infected, it may be suggested that you take a drug called spiramycin for the remainder of your pregnancy. Some women with evidence of recent Toxoplasma infection may already be on spiramycin. Although spiramycin is not effective in treating a baby which is already infected, it may help prevent transmission of the infection. Many of these drugs have side-effects, although these are not experienced by all women. The main problem is that some of these drugs suppress bone marrow function in the baby which is vital to fighting infection, although this has not yet proved to be a serious difficulty. A folic acid supplement may be given (folinic acid) at the same time as the spiramycin to help counteract its side-effects.

At the time of writing, there are calls for universal testing for toxoplasmosis in pregnancy. In theory this might be a good idea, but in practice it won't work. Over 80 per cent of British women test negative (seronegative) for Toxoplasma. The minimum number of tests suggested for continued surveillance throughout pregnancy of a seronegative woman would be three, although some people suggest five. Toxoplasma tests are not yet of sufficient sensitivity and specificity to be foolproof. It is estimated that if universal testing were adopted, 35,000 women in Britain would have a positive first test result; of these, the vast majority would be false positives. More sensitive IgM tests may not be the answer either. The more sensitive the test, the more likely it is that a positive test may reflect infection acquired a year or more ago. At present testing is based on presence of infection rather than handicap and it is simply inappropriate for a mother who has a very low risk of having an affected baby, despite her Toxoplasma infection, to have to be subjected to an invasive procedure of greater risk. Just like the CMV story, all the evidence to date suggests that universal testing for Toxoplasma will cause more deaths of healthy babies than it will prevent births of handicapped babies.

The most important point to make is that if you know your Toxoplasma status is negative before you become pregnant, and then adopt the simplest hygiene measures – things which you should in fact be doing anyway – like washing your hands after gardening, not eating undercooked meat and washing the soil from salads and other vegetables, you have done most of what you need to do to protect your baby. In addition, you should avoid drinking raw goat's milk. By all means have Toxoplasma testing in pregnancy if you really feel it's important to you, (and of course have it if medically indicated) but be aware, you might be submitting yourself to months of needless worry – and still have a perfectly healthy baby.

13   Testing for the Older Mother

To be pregnant is to be subjected to a whirlwind of emotions. What we feel sure about one moment is the very thing that unsettles us with indecision the next. Pregnancy is not an ideal time to be having to make major decisions, yet that is exactly what pregnant women are doing when they consider antenatal testing. Our mothers were perhaps luckier than we are in this regard for they just had babies. But now that the Pandora's box that is antenatal testing is open, what are we, the next generation, to do? Worries about whether to have testing or not are common to all women in pregnancy, but for those women in their late thirties and early forties, there are additional dilemmas.

Health educators sometimes despair of getting health messages through to us, yet one message that has been received loud and clear, and which has been firmly lodged in the national female psyche, is that with increasing maternal age there is an increasing likelihood of having a baby with a chromosomal abnormality such as Down's syndrome. The risk is roughly 1 in 1,000 for a woman aged 27, rising to 1 in 350 by 35, 1 in 100 at 40 and 1 in 25 at 45. A detailed table of risk rates for Down's syndrome is in figure 7 on page 139.

There is something mesmerizing about the word 'risk'. Like a rabbit transfixed by the headlights of a car, we cannot see beyond the word or put it into perspective. A risk of 1 in 100 means that 99 women out of every 100 can expect to have a healthy baby. The 'risk' of Down's may be insignificant in comparison to the risks we run by continuing to smoke during pregnancy or the increased risks we take by not eating properly before or during pregnancy. (See Chapter 3, 'The Risk Ladder'.)

The reasons for the increase in chromosomal disorders with age are to do with cellular ageing. We get our supply of eggs at birth and by the time we get to 35 our eggs are 35 too, and showing their age just as we are. An increase in chromosome abnormalities means not just an increase in the numbers of handicapped babies born to older mothers. It means an increase in the number of fertilized eggs that your body regards as being sub-standard – and that manifests itself as both an increased miscarriage rate and in sub-fertility.

Of course, there are all sorts of reasons why women delay having babies until their thirties. Women marry later these days, they want to have a career first and babies second. They want to feel secure both financially and emotionally before they commit themselves to the responsibilities that a baby brings in its wake. And a major reason for later babies is that women may not have been able to have the baby they wanted when they wanted it.

Women are haunted throughout their lives by the fear that they may be infertile. If you and a friend are both taking the same brand of pill and she gets pregnant and you don't, you quite irrationally decide that perhaps it means, not that she forgot to take it, but that you might not be fertile after all. However, for much of your early reproductive career, you have to put these fears to the back of your mind and just get on with life. And in time, particularly in our twenties, we become seduced by the control that we exercise over our own existence and forget all about fertility for the time being. We reason that if we can switch off pregnancy by using contraception then we will be able to switch it on just as easily when we get around to wanting it in our thirties.

But that's where lots of older women go wrong. It takes the average British couple six months to conceive and it's quite normal for a quarter of all British couples to take at least a year to conceive. However, from the age of 31, women's fertility starts to decline as our bodies begin to have to push out more and more follicle-stimulating hormone to kick-start our ovaries into action. So instead of taking six months, it may take a year – or two years, and all the while our ovaries are in an ever steeper cycle of decline. And here's the dilemma. Older women know that their babies are at greater risk of handicap and that testing is considered advisable in pregnancy but they also know that tests are invasive with a significant risk of spontaneous miscarriage. Above all, they know that it might take even longer to get pregnant next time around. Or that another pregnancy might miscarry anyway. Or that it might not happen at all.

If you fall into this group of women, you may feel that you would rather just know about your baby when it is born and not get on the testing merry-go-round in the first place. You may have already decided before you became pregnant that you would like to opt for either amniocentesis or CVS, and if this is your choice, you will find further details in the relevant chapters. But what if you feel ambivalent about the whole thing?

For a start, let's look at amniocentesis. You may find that it is available in your area to women over 35, while in an adjoining area it is only available to women over 37. Why a woman of 35 can get testing in one area but not in another has little to do with risk rates but everything to do with economics – for while amniocentesis is relatively cheap, karyotyping is not and budgets have to be balanced. About 60–85 per cent of women at risk request an amniocentesis, but this extensive testing of older mothers has resulted in a fall of only 15 per cent in the incidence of Down's syndrome at birth. Several factors are at work here; for instance, some older women may not have been offered an amnio or some may have refused because they have become pregnant following treatment for infertility. There may also be a significant number refusing termination. However, a more potent reason is simply that testing is being offered to a group of women who individually have an increased risk but who collectively account for only a very small proportion of babies born with trisomies such as Down's. In fact, over 60 per cent of Down's babies are born to women who are aged under 35. In short, a great many older women are having amnios because the risk is perceived to be great, when in fact very few Down's babies are actually detected as a result of amnios for maternal age alone.

If amniocentesis doesn't seem to make sense – at least for those just edging into the 'older' age bracket – then CVS would seem to make even less sense for those concerned purely by maternal age. Adding together a miscarriage rate of around 4 per cent and a further 1–2 per cent of cases where there is concern about test accuracy, the case for CVS doesn't stack up in comparison to Down's risk rates of 1 in 100 at age 40.

Anecdotally at least, it would seem that older women are not as concerned about having information about their babies early. Perhaps this is because older women have always known that with amnios and a three to five week wait for results, they would be well into the second trimester of pregnancy before they knew the score. If you are prepared for this well in advance of pregnancy, perhaps you can be relaxed about it. However, this is not to deny how important the greatest advantage of CVS – early results – can be to women, whatever their age. If you feel that early diagnosis is very important to you, then CVS despite its risks is the right choice.

If, however, you are prepared to wait, the ideal scenario for the older woman is perhaps a combination of detailed ultrasound scanning and triple test. The chance that a 40-year-old woman will be found by triple testing to have a Down's syndrome risk under that normally associated with a 35-year-old is a staggering 70 per cent. This would mean having one scan to date your pregnancy at about 16 weeks, followed by triple test. There should be a further detailed fetal anomaly scan at 18–20 weeks, whether or not you have a high risk rate following triple test. If you do have a high risk rate and there is a strong indication of Down's on ultrasound, you will need to confirm this either by amniocentesis or more quickly with cordocentesis. All this could be achieved by 23 weeks, which some women might find unacceptably late both to have confirmation that their baby seems fine or to consider termination.

Of course, as we have seen in all the other chapters on specific procedures, there is still no guarantee of a healthy baby. But such a testing strategy would relieve older women of the worry of causing a very precious pregnancy to miscarry, while holding them in some sort of safety net.

14   Getting an Abnormal Result

While the possibility of getting an abnormal test result is at the back of our minds when we have testing, most of us manage to blot it out imagining that it will never happen to us. This may be reinforced by the experiences of our friends and relatives as the vast majority, if not all, of our particular circle of friends may have had normal test results. It is hardly surprising then that on receiving news of an abnormal test result the first feelings may be ones of shock, numbness and disbelief.

Wondering whether the test result is right, and even disputing it, is a natural first reaction. Karyotyping is not foolproof; 1 in every 1,000 results are false positives. Errors can be made in the complex and exacting task that is DNA analysis; in a series of 659 diagnoses of thalassaemia, for instance, there were 7 errors. But both these examples must be set against the prior risk – 1 in 100 for Down's syndrome at age 40 or 1 in 4 for thalassaemia where both parents are carriers. You may also worry whether results have got muddled up through some ghastly clerical error. Again this is a natural reaction, but everything possible is done to check and double check in laboratories and such errors are incredibly rare.

At least with ultrasound you can be sure that the results are yours and yours alone. However, while there may be no element of doubt about some scan findings, anencephaly for instance, there can be errors in the interpretation of more subtle defects. This is where the experience of the scan operator is the crucial factor. As far as ultrasound diagnosis is concerned, if a condition is diagnosed which might lead you seriously to consider termination of pregnancy, or alternatively which causes you an enormous amount of anxiety, you should seek a second opinion, preferably at a tertiary referral centre or at a centre specializing in fetal medicine (these are listed at the back of the book). In fact, many obstetricians in district general hospitals, although fairly confident of their own diagnosis with ultrasound, will still want to send you to a more experienced centre for confirmation.

Being told of an abnormality discovered on ultrasound scan may in fact be just the beginning of the nightmare, for the finding of one abnormality may indicate the need for further testing. For instance, exomphalos (a condition in which the baby's stomach is outside the abdomen) can be detected with ultrasound and in less severe cases can be successfully corrected with surgery at birth. However, in 30 per cent of cases exomphalos is a marker for chromosome abnormality and therefore diagnosis of exomphalos should be followed by karyotyping (with fetal cells being obtained by cordocentesis) if you are to have the complete picture.

One of your first questions may be 'How badly will my baby be affected?' For some conditions, it will be possible to answer your question with some certainty. For others, all that the obstetrician will be able to do is indicate the parameters of a condition, so that you have some idea of best and worst, but he is unlikely to be able to tell you where your baby fits into this picture. An example might be Down's syndrome where the range of IQs may be anything from 30 to 80, and in which 40 per cent of babies will have heart abnormalities. You may feel that you could cope with a baby with Down's syndrome very happily, no matter what the degree of learning difficulty, but have doubts about the implications of additional major problems such as that likely to be caused by heart disease. Recently, work in Bristol and Nottingham under Professor David James has shown that the baby's behaviour in the womb (how it responds to noise stimuli, etc.) may provide a guide to the extent of likely handicap, although this work is still at an experimental stage.

Positive testing for genetic disease may be similarly afflicted by doubt as to extent of handicap. This is particularly true of dominant gene defects. For instance, in Type 1 neurofibromatosis, although there is complete penetrance of the gene (i.e. it never skips a generation), the effects can be very variable. This is a condition which may be initially diagnosed by the appearance of brown (so-called café au lait) patches in early childhood, which are then followed by soft, fibrous swellings (neurofibromas) on the skin. Beyond this, 75 per cent of those with neurofibromatosis remain unaffected by the complications of the condition such as mental retardation, learning difficulties, seizures and fits. Nothing, apart from a crystal ball, can tell you whether your baby will be among the 75 per cent or the 25 per cent with complications.

Having a clear-cut diagnosis presents enough problems in itself. What many people do not realize is that testing can give you an ambiguous diagnosis. A chromosome count of 46 XYY (a boy with an additional Y chromosome), for instance, results in no abnormality although intelligence may be 10 to 15 points less than that of normal siblings. Now what do you do? Some obstetricians express dismay when faced with couples who wish to terminate a pregnancy following the discovery of an 'abnormal' chromosome finding like this, despite assurances as to likely normality. For the couple involved, the word 'abnormal' may be all that they hear. In addition, they may feel that they cannot live with the uncertainty that such a diagnosis may confer on their lives as they watch their child grow up. However, appropriate counselling before birth can be used to overcome these latter feelings.

The decision about whether to continue with a pregnancy once an abnormality has been determined is one that can be yours and your partner's alone. You may be influenced by many things, by the type of handicap or its extent, by considerations of the family unit you may already have, by your own personal and financial situation, by your likelihood of subsequent pregnancy and so on, but there is no 'right' decision, only what is right for you as an individual, as a couple or as a family. You may feel absolutely sure of your decision or you may feel very ambivalent and this ambivalence may continue, even after you have made your decision. Very many couples, although aware of the love and affection of their family and friends and of the concern of their carers, feel totally alone.

It is not for the obstetrician or for the geneticist to make your decision for you. Their job is to give you as much information – in a clear, objective way – to enable you to make up your own minds and then to support you to the hilt, whatever decision you make. Truly non-directional counselling is probably a myth. Facial expression and even body language may at times say more than any words. The most all counsellors can hope to be is not overtly directive, although there are some situations, where the person being counselled is too young to make an autonomous choice, when directive counselling is helpful.

Your obstetrician sees your predicament, understands your hurt and your feelings of being both in control of events and yet totally out of control. He or she will be happy to direct you to other sources of expertise if you feel that this might be helpful, such as doctors specializing in the type of problem that your baby has, or other families who have been through the same thing. It is worth saying that this process of gathering information may be important to you in the future, when you will at least feel that you made your decision with all possible information to hand. You may just feel overwhelmed by it all, asking your doctor 'What would you do?' in the hope that, by answering, he or she will make your decision for you. Most counsellors won't be drawn on this question, although they probably will tell you what other couples in the same situation have done.

Very often, what you thought about termination prior to

pregnancy flies out of the window completely – about 30 per cent of termination decisions are contrary to previous conviction not to terminate. There might be an equal percentage the other way. Now it is just you and your baby – not a hypothetical moral dilemma but the real thing, which has not just a considered, decided and then immediately forgotten conclusion, but one with lifelong implications.

Once the initial shock has passed, there will be feelings of overwhelming sadness and loss not only because the baby you wanted, which you and your friends and family expected shortly to welcome into the world is not as you had hoped, but also because, if you decide to terminate, you will be losing your baby as well. You may feel relief that you have found out 'in time'. You may wish you had never had testing at all and had never found out. You may feel angry – 'Why did it have to happen to me?' Above all, there may be considerable feelings of guilt – that your baby's condition is somehow your fault, that you must have done something during your pregnancy to make it happen or that in some way you are being punished, through your child, for some misdemeanour. It is particularly common for women who have had previous terminations on social grounds to feel like this. While such feelings are natural, they, like many of the feelings of guilt, are without foundation. It is all too easy in this distressing situation to make accusations, to shoot the messenger in the foot and then to direct your anger and hurt at your partner. He may find the burden equally intolerable and while he may try to be there for you, he too is experiencing grief.

Deciding to have the baby

As outlined in Chapter 2, 'To Test or Not to Test', diagnosis of abnormality is emphatically not automatically linked to termination. For many women, discovery of abnormality may be the first realization that their baby will be different and that he or she will need a great deal of special care and attention, the foundations of which must be laid before birth. For some women, discovery of a lethal handicap such as anencephaly may mark the beginning of a period of preparation leading up to the birth of a baby that they wanted to greet into the world, to hold and touch and then allow to die in their arms. A decision to go on requires as much courage, faith and support from family and friends as does a decision to terminate a pregnancy. Neither is easy. Sometimes women find that while they want to go ahead, their partner does not. This can be a source of the greatest hurt. Finding an alternative source of support is essential – your minister may be able to help, or a support group such as LIFE.

HAVING A TERMINATION

Termination of pregnancy prior to the time when the baby is considered viable is legal if continuation of pregnancy would involve a greater risk to the mother's life, to the mother's physical or mental health or the existing child(ren)'s health. The legally defined limit of viability is now 24 weeks (having been recently reduced from 28 weeks). When the legislation (The Abortion Act 1967, as amended by the Human Fertilization and Embryology Act 1990) was being drawn up, there was awareness that diagnosis of abnormality might, for many good reasons, not be made until after 24 weeks, therefore a time limit for termination for 'substantial risk of serious handicap' was not imposed. There is now in effect no upper limit; in other words termination of pregnancy because of 'substantial risk of serious handicap' could occur up to 40 weeks. I make this point because when a diagnosis of abnormality is made, parents sometimes assume that termination must take place quickly because of 'the law'. This is not the case.

Once diagnosis has been confirmed and you have decided to have a termination, there is a tendency 'to get it over with', with appointments for admission to hospital being made the next morning, or even the same day. While some couples might feel that waiting to be admitted is a trial in itself, to be avoided at all costs, there are other couples who need to take time, both to prepare themselves mentally for the ordeal ahead and to some extent to come to terms with their own feelings. A day, a week or even two weeks will make no difference. Your obstetrician will understand if you would prefer to wait and some even advise waiting a day or two. However, he will be happy to accede to your wishes either way.

Practicalities You will need to be admitted to hospital. A second trimester termination under general anaesthetic will involve at least an overnight stay. An induced labour may take longer. If you have other children, you need to make appropriate arrangements for them. You will need all the usual things for a hospital visit – nightdress, wash things and so on, as well as sanitary towels, small change for telephones and perhaps something to eat. There is nothing so awful as you and your partner being hungry as well as miserable during those interminable early morning hours when you may not have eaten for ages, but when everywhere is shut. You might also decide at this stage what you are going to tell your friends and whether you want visitors. Some friends may want to send flowers but if you think that you will find this too upsetting, it is worth saying so in advance. Hospitals will make every effort to put women in a single ward, rather than on the general antenatal ward, if they can. You may on the other hand prefer to be with other women and if you do, say so.

First trimester termination

This will be undertaken under general anaesthetic using a vacuum aspiration technique and it will usually be possible to do this as an outpatient procedure.

Second trimester termination

Discovery of fetal abnormality in the first trimester of pregnancy is probably the exception rather than the rule. Only those with specific risk factors prior to pregnancy, such as maternal age or a family history of genetic disease, will have access to methods of diagnosis such as CVS or early amniocentesis which are used in the first trimester. For many women, the first inkling that anything may be amiss comes after the 16th week of pregnancy, when the fetal anomaly scan is usually undertaken, or a little after this when the results of triple test screening come through, or at about 20 weeks, when the results of conventionally timed amniocentesis are available. For some women, results may come even later. If a woman opts for termination at this stage, outpatient techniques such as vacuum aspiration are no longer an option. Instead, you will have to go through a process which will be very similar to a full term labour. You will need to stay in hospital, at least overnight or longer, depending on how long the procedure takes and how you are feeling. Under the terms of the amended Abortion Act, all terminations after 24 weeks have to be carried out in an NHS hospital. A very small number of private hospitals are also licensed to undertake late terminations and the British Pregnancy Advisory Service can provide details of these.

A prostaglandin infusion is probably the most commonly used method of termination in Britain. Prostaglandins are natural hormone–like substances which were first described in 1935, following their discovery in seminal fluid. They were subsequently found to be involved in the mechanism of labour and to cause contractions of the womb. Prostaglandins can be given to a woman either intra- or extra-amniotically or as vaginal pessaries, depending on the stage of pregnancy.

More than one vaginal pessary may have to be used and these are given at intervals over a 24-hour period. Extra-amniotic introduction of prostaglandins involves the insertion of a small tube into the cervix. The tube is attached to a pump which initially delivers about 1–2 ml an hour of fluid (a salt solution containing prostaglandins). The volume of fluid may gradually be increased. Alternatively prostaglandins can be injected into the amniotic sac which surrounds the baby. A long fine needle is used to do this, which will be guided by ultrasound. With all these methods, it will take several hours for contractions to begin. You may feel sick or have diarrhoea. Severe nausea can be countered by taking anti-nausea drugs, either as tablets or in injection form. If the waiting period is too long, you may also be given another drug, oxytocin (brand name, Syntocinon), to further stimulate contractions. This drug is given as an intravenous drip.

At first contractions will feel like period cramps but they will get progressively more painful. Contractions are not usually as strong as those of term labour but they can still cause a great deal of pain. Adequate pain relief is essential, usually either as injections or possibly an epidural but you should ask about this before the procedure begins. Women often ask why they can't just have a general anaesthetic, rather than go through such an unpleasant experience fully conscious. The answer is that the procedure is too lengthy (12 to 24 hours over all) for a general anaesthetic to be used safely. There is, unfortunately, no way of making it shorter, at least not without causing damage to your cervix, and thereby putting future pregnancies at risk of late miscarriage or premature delivery.

As in normal labour, at some point you will experience a

gushing of liquid – this is the amniotic sac bursting, releasing the fluid. After several hours of contractions, the baby will be expelled, followed shortly afterwards by the placenta. You may be given an injection of the hormone oxytocin to help the womb contract back to its pre-pregnancy place in your pelvis.

Sometimes the placenta does not come away completely and you may then need to have this removed by curettage (scraping with a knife) under general anaesthetic, straight after termination.

When prostaglandins alone are used, usually between 12 and 20 weeks, the baby may be born alive and may show signs of life for a few minutes before dying. Because at later stages of pregnancy the baby might, against all odds, survive despite its handicap, later terminations usually use the intra-amniotic method of infusing prostaglandin. At the same time, an injection of urea will be put into the amniotic sac and this will kill the baby as well as help to initiate contractions. Practice, however, varies quite widely across the country. Some centres prefer to inject 2–3 ml of potassium chloride directly into the baby's heart or a bubble of air into the baby's circulation, using a needle guided by ultrasound, causing death instantly. You may well feel very squeamish reading this but there isn't any other way of putting it – the purpose of termination is, after all, that a baby dies and a lethal injection is probably the quickest and surest way of doing this.

After the birth, you may want to see or hold the baby and to take some photographs for yourself. The hospital will almost certainly want to take medical photographs for your records and these may be very important for future genetic counselling. The fear of what your baby may look like is sometimes a lot worse than the reality. Many babies with quite severe degrees of abnormality will look quite normal. You may want other things by which you can remember your baby, such as a foot- or hand-print. You may want to be alone with your baby and staff will try to ensure that you have a room where you can be quiet and comfortable for as long as you want to be. After a while, your baby's body will begin to feel cold and rigid, but wrapping him or her in a shawl may make holding feel more natural. You may want to dress your baby perhaps in a way that makes the disability less obvious. It is important to say that the body will not deteriorate and you will not be asked to part with your baby until you are both ready. Your baby's body will usually be kept for a stated period of time, so that if you want to see her or him again, you can. You will not have to go to the mortuary; a member of staff will bring the baby to you. You may want to name the baby. For many couples, their religious faith may become especially important at this time, offering comfort and hope. Even those with no previously expressed religious beliefs may feel the need to talk to the hospital chaplain or to have the time and space in which to say their own private prayers. You may want the baby to be blessed either by the hospital chaplain or some other religious person.

After 24 weeks' gestation, sometimes the baby can be certified as having been born alive, thus providing parents with both a birth and death certificate. This may not, however, always happen and a stillbirth certificate may be provided instead.

POST MORTEM

There is no obligation on parents to have a post mortem and parental consent is required for one. You may feel that you already know the diagnosis, but a post mortem examination of the baby may reveal additional information about the nature of the handicapping condition which will have implications for future pregnancies and for this reason a post mortem is immensely important. For instance, other abnormalities not seen on scan may be detected which may alter the diagnosis if not the prognosis of your baby's condition. In a recent study over five years, the pre-termination diagnosis was modified in 53 of 133 babies aborted after findings of abnormality of scans. In some cases the modified diagnosis led to an increased risk of recurrence, in others a decreased risk. Terminations may be scheduled to take place when a full complement of pathology staff is available to undertake an immediate post mortem (i.e. not at a weekend or on a bank holiday). Sometimes this may mean waiting and although this may be difficult and possibly cause distress, it is best practice.

An unspoken fear among some couples is what they would do if a post mortem revealed that, after all, their baby had been normal. A post mortem result will generally be used to amplify and confirm a diagnosis. It will never be used to undermine the parents but the discovery that a baby does not have what was originally diagnosed has major implications for your next pregnancy. It may be very difficult to cope with, but it may also bring a sense of relief.

Parents also fear the damage that may be done to their baby by the post mortem. The post mortem technicians will take the greatest possible care to restore the baby and to dress it carefully. This may of course be more difficult, although not impossible, at earlier gestations.

Deciding whether or not to have a funeral is an entirely personal decision and one which need not necessarily be related to gestational age. If you have decided not to have a funeral, you can ask the hospital to dispose of your baby's body after the post mortem. You will need to be reassured that this is done in a respectful way – some hospitals, for instance, suggest incineration following a short committal service conducted by the hospital chaplain.

Having a post mortem should not necessarily mean that a funeral has to be delayed. For parents of some religious faiths it is important that the funeral should take place as soon as possible, usually within 24 hours. If you decide to have a funeral, you will need a letter from the hospital authorizing the release of your baby's body once the post mortem has been completed. You may feel that although you want a funeral, you cannot cope with the arrangements yourself and may need to ask someone else to do it, perhaps a close friend.

Alternative Techniques of Termination

Dilatation and evacuation is a newer method of second trimester termination which combines a D & C and vacuum aspiration techniques. It is much quicker, but it requires specialist expertise (currently fewer than half a dozen gynaecologists in London are able to use it, although you should find it available at all fetal medicine centres in Britain) and is only suitable up to 24 weeks. The cervix is first softened (usually with a prostaglandin) and then later, under general anaesthetic, the cervix is gradually dilated. The baby receives, under ultrasound guidance, a lethal dose of potassium chloride directly into the heart and thereafter embryotomy is necessary (breaking the baby up) in order to remove it and the placenta, piecemeal, through the cervix. Careful ultrasound control ensures that no products of conception remain in the womb. Evidently there is no baby to see afterwards and some parents may find that this may make the grieving process more difficult. Dilatation and evacuation involves less emotional distress than the prolonged and painful process following the medical induction of labour. The only indication for not undertaking this procedure is to obtain an intact baby in order to allow careful post mortem evaluation for the diagnosis of a specific structural abnormality.

AFTERWARDS

One of the most distressing things about losing a baby is that your body goes on just as if there were still a baby. Soon after the termination your breasts will begin to swell and throb and to leak milk. It is a very painful reminder of your loss. You may be prescribed drugs to suppress lactation or be asked to express some milk gently (but not enough to overstimulate your breasts) to ease your discomfort. Pain relief, a good bra and cold compresses may help but you should be prepared, in the absence of drug treatment, for milk to continue to be produced for several days or even a couple of weeks, depending on the stage of pregnancy at which you had the termination. You will also experience bleeding for some days if not weeks afterwards.

Coping

While some couples prefer to keep news of the diagnosis or of their decision to terminate the pregnancy to themselves, others will tell a close family member or a couple of special friends. Sharing your hurt and grief may be very beneficial but sometimes couples say afterwards that 'nobody offered any help' when they spoke to them. This may represent an unrealistic expectation of what friends or family can do when you tell them news of this sort. They are not trained counsellors. They will be almost as shocked by the news as you are. They may feel powerless to help, with the words that they speak not necessarily being what they really feel but merely an automatic pilot response – things like 'cheer up' or 'don't take it so badly' or 'it's all for the best'.

If you have relatives or friends in this situation, practical support may be of the greatest help to both you and them – at least you can feel that you are doing something positive, although in reality by just listening you may already be giving the best and most positive form of support. Trauma such as this uses up extraordinary amounts of energy, both emotional and physical, exhausting couples and leaving nothing for the day-to-day practicalities of life. Looking after other children if there are any, doing minor domestic chores such as lawn mowing, shopping, ironing or even just the hoovering and dusting, without necessarily being asked to do so but without being intrusive either, will be very helpful. Don't be offended, however, if the couple do not notice at the time whether you have their ironing or not – much of their daily life will just pass them by in a blur for a while, so overwhelming is their trauma.

This complete exhaustion of physical and emotional resources may have other implications. One half of a couple may accomplish the grieving process painfully but adequately, but have no resources left to interact effectively with, let alone be supportive to his or her partner. In this way common and normal feelings of guilt, anger and of accusation (however irrational) may become magnified and transmitted to the partner, causing a deterioration in the relationship.

Very often attention in these situations is directed to the mother, because of the implicit understanding of the mother/ baby bond and the assumption that the mother will suffer most. Traditionally the man is expected to be strong and supportive of his partner. It may be particularly difficult for the father to declare his need for support and advice, especially if he is young and relatively inexperienced, but he needs it too.

Telling other people can be very difficult. Some couples prefer to say that the pregnancy has ended in a miscarriage or stillbirth rather than tell the truth. This is entirely understandable. There may be disapproval, particularly from those who have strong religious convictions and it is particularly painful if this attitude comes from your own parents, resulting in a strained relationship for some time. It is easy to assume if people seem to avoid you that they also do not approve but it may simply be that they just do not know what to say to you.

If you have other children, it will help if you tell them what has happened. Of course what you tell them will depend on their age and their level of understanding but not telling them can lead them to believe that something has happened which is so dreadful that you can't tell them. This may frighten them. Above all else, it is important to reassure children that they are not to blame in any way. It might be helpful to tell your child's teacher or playgroup leader what has happened. Another reassurance for your child, which may seem obvious, is that the thing that killed your baby will not kill him or her too.

Children differ in their reactions to news of this kind. They can be utterly heartless, even cross with you because you aren't going to give them the baby brother or sister they thought they were going to have. They may be incredibly sweet and understanding. I had a miscarriage because of a chromosome abnormality. I knew from an early stage that the pregnancy was not going to reach full term and was relieved rather than sad when the miscarriage finally happened. But when I told my four-year-old and he just said, 'I love you, Mummy', and started to cry himself, that was the end, the floodgates opened and the two of us just sat there howling like a couple of puppies. It was the best thing that could have happened for both of us.

One of the most difficult things after an experience like this is that you may find your friends stop telling you baby news, or bringing their new babies to see you, because they think it will upset you. This can be very isolating. You may well be sad but it doesn't stop you being happy for other people, so you may have to take the initiative in making it known that you don't mind. On the other hand, you may find it incredibly difficult to be near babies for a while.

If things get too much, if you feel you are being a burden to your friends or can't share what you feel with them, try ringing an organization such as SATFA (Support after Termination for Abnormality) or CARE if you live in Scotland. Not only will they understand what you are going through, but more importantly they will be able to put you in touch with someone else who has experienced the same thing. Knowing that you are not the only person in the world to be going through this can be of immense comfort.

One further point to make is that although support services in hospitals may be good, the same often cannot be said of primary care services. Normally, the mother of any baby born alive or dead after 28 weeks would have statutory visits from a midwife, health visitor, etc. Following a termination for abnormality such support rarely appears, even though you may have many of the same concerns and symptoms as these other women. In particular, you may feel, in addition to your grief, a bout of 'baby blues' three or four days after the termination, when you feel desperately weepy and miserable.

Feelings of guilt may continue for a very long period of time. In addition to the guilt at having been the direct cause of your baby's death, there are other feelings of guilt which may come in a later, more reflective phase. Prior to the finding of a genetic abnormality, most couples will not have considered themselves defective and will have expected an ideal or at least a normal family. With a diagnosis of abnormality, a new dimension of personal self and family self has to be confronted which is perceived as deficient and defective. The adjustment needed to integrate and bring back into equilibrium the ideal self and the perceived self is part of the grief process following discovery of abnormality. The process may be made more difficult by attributions of blame to one partner or the other, as being the bearer of the defective gene. In many cases this is pointless speculation – both parents are biologically responsible for their baby. But in some conditions there may be no doubt which parent carried the abnormal gene. The reality is that we all carry defective genes. Most of us are lucky in that the 'normal' copy of our genes prevents us coming to any harm. Many couples may have had two, three or even more children, all healthy, without ever discovering through the birth of an affected child that they were both carriers of a recessive gene.

15   Genetic Counselling

It will usually take about six weeks to get all the results through after the post mortem and this is the time at which you are likely to be given an appointment to discuss them with your obstetrician or alternatively a geneticist.

Wherever possible, individuals should be offered genetic counselling at a genetic clinic. While genetic advice may sometimes be given by GPs or obstetricians, advice by a specialist is always preferable. This is partly because of the very large number of inherited conditions, most of which are rare. It is not uncommon for obstetricians or GPs to have seldom if ever seen a similar case to yours before. Modes of inheritance, as we saw in earlier chapters, can be very complex – with alternative modes of inheritance in the same condition or conditions which are part hereditary and part environmental. At the end of the day, what parents want is a figure for risk recurrence and this very often involves the study of up-to-date literature, which can be very extensive.

Geneticists must be the only doctors to have no beds allocated to their speciality. Because of their lack of visibility, at least in terms of hospital beds, specialist genetic services are sometimes not accorded the importance they deserve. Although diseases of wholly genetic origin are often individually rare, they are numerous, incurable and often severe in their effects, accounting for one-third of admissions to paediatric wards alone. Genetic counselling covers more than estimating risks and extends beyond the person affected by genetic disease, to his or her whole family, in changing situations over many years. The first job of the clinical geneticist is to establish an accurate diagnosis on which to base counselling and then to provide information about prognosis and follow-up, the risk of developing or transmitting the disorder and the ways in which this might be prevented or ameliorated. Throughout, the whole family requires support in adjusting to the implications of genetic disease and the consequent decisions that have to be made. Incorrect counselling by well-meaning but ill-informed, non-specialist doctors can be devastating in its impact and the importance of seeking advice from one of the regional genetic centres listed at the back of this book, even for so-called common problems, cannot be overstated. It is worth quoting from a recent report, 'Clinical genetic services in 1990 and beyond' by the Royal College of Physicians: 'Genetic counselling should be regarded as a procedure comparable to surgical operations and to medication in both its potential for healing but also for harm when the consequences may extend through several lifetimes.'

Your first visit to a geneticist may be for a diagnosis of the problem that affected your baby, or you may already know the diagnosis but want specialist advice. More likely still, you may have a family history of genetic disease. The appointment is likely to take place in a quiet and comfortable room, far from the hustle and bustle of normal hospital life. You will probably spend at least an hour, perhaps two, on your first visit, and be offered further appointments depending on your need. An important thing to say at the outset is that most couples, especially if they are still reeling from the shock of discovering abnormality, are not able to take in much information on their first visit. Often at the end of your appointment, you will be given written information about your particular condition, if it is a common one, and asked to return. On your second visit you may have many more questions and be able, having read and re-read any information leaflets in the interim, to take on board a great deal more of what you may be told.

The first requirement is an accurate diagnosis. This may not be straightforward because genetic disease can be very variable, with different members of a family with the same disorder seeing different specialists with a range of symptoms all resulting from the same problem. Furthermore, the person requesting genetic counselling may not be the one affected and the diagnosis may have to be confirmed by examining the affected relative or reviewing their hospital records.

As far as having had a baby with an abnormality is concerned, the most important first step is to establish exactly what problem your baby had. This is not always easy. The geneticist will have gathered together clinical photographs, X rays and post mortem results prior to your visit. Your baby may have had 'dysmorphic' features – that is, a combination of facial and other features which constitute a slight or great departure from the normal shape and appearance. Many dysmorphic syndromes are genetic but tracking down the exact syndrome, when many of them have shared characteristics, requires patience and considerable skill. But combining such skill with results of cytogenetic analysis and pathological examination will provide as accurate a diagnosis as possible.

DRAWING UP A FAMILY PEDIGREE

Giving an assessment of risk for a subsequent pregnancy depends on the mode of inheritance of the condition diagnosed. As part of the genetic counselling session, a family tree or pedigree will be drawn up. A range of special symbols are used which simplify the recording of what may be quite complex information. Usually the counsellor will start by recording the pregnancies of the mother with their outcome, then list her brothers and sisters, living or dead, together with her mother's stillbirths or miscarriages if known. The children of her brothers and sisters (sibs) are then filled in. Enquiries will be made about her father and mother, uncles, aunts and cousins, together with the catch-all question, does she know anything that might be relevant about them?

Most of our hearsay medical record-keeping is far from accurate. Is an aunt saying 'Your cousin Vic was a bit odd' a diagnosis of mental handicap or was he just given to stripping his bike down in the bedroom? Different attitudes to illness in the past and the tendency of an older generation not to talk about 'problems' can leave large gaps in the knowledge about the rest of the family's health. It wasn't until after a relative's death that my uncle, a solicitor, had occasion to review my grandfather's will. He discovered to his astonishment that there had been six children in the family, not five as had always been believed. The last child, a girl born in 1898, had been placed in an institution at an early age. At that time she was still alive (although all her brothers and sisters were dead) and, my uncle discovered, in the same institution – some 70 years or so on. Her handicap? She had been born profoundly deaf.

Often it may be necessary for the geneticist to request medical records from other members of the family. The one certain aspect of a genetic disease is that it is a family disorder. There are parents who may be critical, there may be brothers and sisters who are convinced that they too carry the gene but who hope against hope that they do not. There are copers in the family and there are the black sheep – the ones who won't admit that genetic illness is present and won't talk to a doctor, or indeed to anyone else. The geneticist may have to do more than just create a family pedigree. He may have to empathize with relatives whose points of view may be unclear or even hostile.

ASSESSMENT OF RISK

Genetic risks are assessed in terms of probabilities. They range from a very big risk of 1 in 2 with a dominant gene, or 1 in 4 with a recessive gene, through a range of decreasing risks which may ultimately reach very low levels indeed. Sometimes risk assessment is straightforward. In other cases, risk may vary depending on the number of relatives also affected. Although this is a sweeping generalization, it is the least complicated transmissions – where the father or mother has a dominant condition, for instance – that give the really bad chances, while every further complication of the genetic scheme reduces the proportion of affected persons among relatives.

What constitutes risk?

In general risks fall into two groups: those that are worse than 1 in 10 and those that are better than 1 in 20. There are very few intermediate figures. Couples usually need some sort of yardstick against which they can measure their risk and the one that is usually given is the chance of any random pregnancy ending with a baby with some form of handicapping condition which is 1 in 40. If a risk is better than 1 in 20, a repeat tragedy in pregnancy is as likely to be a result of a totally different condition as of the problem for which counselling is being sought. Obviously a great deal depends on the nature of the condition and certainly amniocentesis or another form of testing would still be indicated.

Consanguinity

Consanguinity – the relationship by blood – can significantly affect the assessment of genetic risk. Marriage between first cousins generally increases the risk of severe abnormality and mortality in offspring by 5 per cent, compared with that in the general population. Marriage between first- and second-degree relatives (sisters and brothers, first cousins) is almost universally illegal, although marriages between uncles and nieces are not unknown in Asian countries. Marriage between third-degree relatives is very common in Asian cultures and is well documented among Asian families living in Britain. The offspring of incestuous relationships are at high risk of abnormality with only half of the children born to first-degree relatives being normal.

Genetic registers

Genetic centres compile and keep genetic registers. These list all people at risk of developing or transmitting a particular disorder so that counselling can be offered. A register allows individuals to be followed up over a long period of time, which is particularly important for children at risk who will not need counselling for antenatal diagnosis for many years to come. Registers are of supreme importance in one other respect. I have already indicated that DNA analysis is advancing at an incredible pace. It is quite possible that conditions for which DNA analysis was not possible during pregnancy may be the subject of new methods of diagnosis within a couple of years. Being able to contact a woman directly and tell her about this new advance, thus allowing her to proceed with a pregnancy that she might not previously have attempted, is very important. Registers can also provide data on the incidence of disease and the effect of counselling or preventive programmes. All genetic registers are held on computer and are subject to the Data Protection Act. No one is included in a register without having given prior informed consent.

If you are seeing a geneticist prior to pregnancy because you already know that there is an inherited disease in your family, a family history will be taken in the same way that I have already described.

There are several difficult ethical problems which arise in relation to genetic services. For instance, the issue of paternity is one that may present the geneticist with special concerns. It is certainly not unknown for genetic tests to reveal that the supposed father is not the real father of the child. Such information is strictly confidential and mothers need not worry that their secret will be revealed. However, the geneticist may ask the mother to consider telling the father, if only because otherwise he will believe that he is the carrier of a genetic disease when in fact he is not. Sometimes a geneticist in this situation may claim that the condition is a new mutation not carried by the father in an attempt to find a compromise between confidentiality and the need to let a third party have correct information.

If the issues related to non-paternity are difficult, there are others which are even thornier, for instance, situations where relatives are in a position to refuse testing, thereby preventing access to the relevant information. There is no law which allows coercion of reluctant relatives, even though there is a precedent in law for production of biological samples, for instance, in cases of suspected drinking and driving. Even more difficult is the situation where a GP or other doctor has access to samples (for instance, a blood sample taken for an entirely different reason) which could theoretically be tested for the genetic condition for which a patient has previously refused testing. Should the doctor carry out the genetic testing required without his patient's knowledge?

Linkage studies

Sometimes other tests besides the presence or absence of symptoms of a disease can be important in predicting transmission of a gene, particularly in late onset diseases such as Huntington's chorea. Linkage studies are studies of genes that are known to be closely linked, in terms of physical location, to genes that cause disease. One such linkage study is that of the ability to secrete a chemical called ABH into the saliva and myotonic dystrophy. Knowledge of secretor status may not give the whole answer to the question, 'Will I (or my baby) have this disease?' but it can reduce (or increase) probabilities.

As those who wrote the RCP report so wisely said, genetic counselling is akin to surgery. It can be devastating in its impact – but if handled properly, by those with the greatest experience, it can provide the clearest of information, casting at least some light on a very difficult situation.

16 Directory

SINGLE GENE DISORDERS

More than 5,000 human single gene defects have already been recognized, affecting about 1 per cent of the population. Between 13,000 and 20,000 babies with single gene defects are born each year.

For some conditions prenatal testing is possible and, where applicable, this is indicated. Because of the pace of change in the field of genetics at present, it may well be that although prenatal testing was not possible at the time of writing, the situation will have changed by the time you read this book. Couples should check with a regional genetics centre, or alternatively the appropriate specialist support group. The approximate incidence of each condition has been given; however, expert sources vary quite widely in their estimates of incidence and once again you would be best seeking up-to-date specialist advice. The variation in incidence arises because single gene defects often share symptoms, which may have resulted in the past, before more sophisticated gene technology was available, in some conditions being incorrectly attributed.

Where carrier testing is indicated as being available, the most usual method of testing would involve taking a blood sample, although for some carrier testing, such as that for cystic fibrosis, a simple mouthwash is all that is required. Pre- and post-test counselling would form an essential part of such carrier testing.

ACHONDROPLASIA

A type of dwarfism, with short limbs and normal length trunk. Maximum adult height for boys is 132 cm and 123 cm for girls. Normal intelligence and lifespan. Incidence is 1 in 26,000 live births.

> Autosomal dominant but can arise as a new mutation; linked to increasing paternal age.
> Detection: ultrasound.
> Support group: The Child Growth Foundation, 2 Mayfield Avenue, Chiswick, W4 1PW 081-995 0257

CONGENITAL ADRENAL HYPERPLASIA

This uncommon disorder (1 in 17,000 births) is also called virilizing adrenal hyperplasia. The gene defect causes variable enzyme deficiencies which block the production of hydrocortisone and aldosterone (the hormone involved in the balance of salt and water in the body) and also affects the sex hormones. Prompt treatment with replacement hormones means that affected babies live a normal healthy life.

> Autosomal recessive. Carrier detection possible.
> Prenatal diagnosis by assay of amniotic fluid, and by gene analysis using CVS and amniocentesis.

CONGENITAL SPHEROCYTOSIS

A condition in which there is a large number of unusually small, round red blood cells (spherocytes) in the circulation. These cells are fragile and have a much reduced lifespan because they are readily trapped, broken up and destroyed when they pass through the spleen. Red cell destruction may exceed the formation of new red blood cells, resulting in anaemia. Hereditary spherocytosis is the most common form of inherited anaemia in people of Northern European extraction, occurring in the UK in about 1 in 4,500 people. Removal of the spleen usually leads to dramatic and sometimes permanent improvement in health, although there is a subsequent increased susceptibility to infection.

Autosomal dominant.

CYSTIC FIBROSIS

The most common genetic disease in the UK, with 1 in 20 people being a carrier. CF affects 1 in every 1,500 babies born in the UK. The disease is characterized by a tendency to chronic lung infections and an inability to absorb fats and other nutrients from food. It is also called mucoviscidosis because of the secretion of a sticky (viscid) mucus which then causes obstruction in the nose, throat, airways and intestines. The introduction of a new range of antibiotic drugs has meant that most CF sufferers now survive into adult life, although CF remains a serious and potentially fatal disorder. Treatment is with daily physiotherapy, antibiotics to combat respiratory infections and additions of enzyme supplements to the diet. Heart-lung and lung transplants have been undertaken with encouraging results.

The gene that causes CF has been isolated and is located on Chromosome 7. At the time of writing a national carrier screening programme is under discussion.

Autosomal recessive. Carrier screening.

Prenatal diagnosis using amniocentesis or CVS.

Support group: Cystic Fibrosis Research Trust,

Alexandra House, Bromley Road, Bromley, Kent 081-464 7211

CYSTINURIA

A disease in which there is increased urine output and reduced intestinal absorption of some amino acids resulting in recurrent kidney stones. Incidence is 1 in 10,000 and with treatment those affected lead a normal life.

> Autosomal recessive. Carrier detection possible.
> Prenatal diagnosis using CVS or, preferably,
> amniocentesis.

FRIEDRICH'S ATAXIA

A condition with an incidence of 1 in 50,000 in which degeneration of nerve fibres in the spinal cord causes ataxia (loss of co-ordinated movement and balance). The disease becomes progressively more severe with half of the sufferers confined to a wheelchair within ten years of onset. Death generally occurs in the third decade.

> Autosomal recessive. Carrier detection.
> Prenatal diagnosis using CVS.
> Support group: Friedrich's Ataxia, Copse Edge,
> Thursley Road, Elstead, Godalming, Surrey GU8 6DJ
> 0252-702864

GILLES DE LA TOURETTE SYNDROME

A condition which causes motor and vocal tics. There may also be compulsive or obsessive behaviour and learning difficulties. About half the sufferers have episodes of coprolalia (using foul language).

> Autosomal dominant.
> No prenatal diagnosis available.
> Support group: Tourette Syndrome (UK) Association,
> 169 Wickham Street, Welling, Kent DA16 3BS
> 081-304 5446

HAEMOPHILIA

A bleeding disorder caused by a deficiency of a blood protein, Factor VIII. Haemophilia is a sex-linked disease in which affected men may pass the defective gene on to none of their sons but to all of their daughters, who will be carriers. Some of their daughters' sons will be affected and some of their daughters will be carriers. The severity of the disorder differs markedly in those affected. In the most severe cases bleeding into joints may cause deformities of the ankles, knees and other joints. Treatment is possible by transfusions of concentrates containing Factor VIII. The incidence of haemophilia A is 1 in 5,000 men; for haemophilia B (Christmas disease) it is 1 in 30,000 men.

> X-linked recessive (although spontaneous mutations do occur).
> Prenatal diagnosis by DNA analysis following CVS, or by fetal sexing followed by cordocentesis to measure fetal levels of Factor VIII.
> Support group: The Haemophilia Society, 123 Westminster Bridge Road, London SE1 7HR
> 071-928 2020

HUNTINGTON'S CHOREA

A disease in which degeneration of nerve cell clusters in the brain results in chorea (rapid, jerky movements) and dementia. Symptoms do not usually appear until mid-life. Incidence is 1 in 18,000 in the UK. Both men and women are affected. In some cases where detailed family history is available, predictive testing is possible, although extensive counselling is required both before and after such a test. There is a diagnostic error rate of 2 per cent.

> Autosomal dominant. Carrier testing.
> Prenatal diagnosis using amniocentesis or CVS.

Support group: Huntington's Disease Association,
108 Battersea High Street, London SW11 3HP
071-223 7000

HYPERCHOLESTEROLAEMIA, FAMILIAL

A disease in which a protein responsible for removing cholesterol from the blood is defective. Resulting high levels of
blood cholesterol make affected individuals susceptible to early
heart disease. Without treatment 50 per cent of affected men
will be dead by the age of 60 and this condition accounts for
about 8 per cent of early ischaemic heart disease in men.

Autosomal dominant or co-dominant. Presymptomatic
diagnosis using pedigrees.
Prenatal diagnosis possible via CVS or amniocentesis.
Support group: The Family Heart Association, PO Box
116, Kidlington, Oxford OX5 2DH 086-75 0292

INTESTINAL POLYPOSIS (also known as familial polyposis)

A condition in which there are numerous (often more than
1,000) polyps in the colon and rectum. Without preventive
treatment (a colectomy) the development of cancer of the
colon by the age of 40 is almost certain. There are three
different types and their combined frequency is about 1 in
10,000.

Autosomal dominant.
Prenatal diagnosis for Types I and III via CVS or
amniocentesis.

LESCH-NYAN SYNDROME

A condition affecting 1 in 10,000 males. Abnormal levels of
uric acid are produced and red blood cells are also affected,

causing progressive spasticity and blindness in infancy with mental retardation, kidney stones and gouty arthritis.

> X-linked recessive trait. Carrier testing.
> Prenatal diagnosis by testing sample of fetal blood obtained by cordocentesis.

MARFAN SYNDROME

A disorder of connective tissue which results in abnormalities of the skeleton, heart and eyes. Incidence is about 1 in 50,000. Typical Marfan sufferers are very tall and thin, with long spidery fingers. The chest and spine are often deformed.

> Autosomal dominant with 15 per cent of cases being mutations.
> Prenatal diagnosis not possible.
> Support group: Marfan Association, 6 Queen's Road, Farnborough, Hants GU14 6DH 0252-547441

MUCOPOLYSACCHARIDOSES

There are four main types, Hurler syndrome (gargoylism), Hunter syndrome, Sanfilippo syndrome and Morquio disease. Each is characterized by lack of a specific enzyme which results in an abnormal accumulation of substances known as muco-polysaccharides in the tissues. Physical and mental growth is affected. There may also be cardiac and skeletal abnormalities. Death takes place in either the second or third decade. Combined frequency is 1 in 20,000 with Sanfilippo being the most common type.

> Autosomal recessive except for Hunter disease which is X-linked. Carrier detection.
> Prenatal diagnosis by analysis of amniotic fluid or by enzyme assay in cells obtained via CVS.
> Support group: The Society for Mucopolysaccharide

Diseases, 7 Chessfield Park, Little Chalfont, Bucks
0494-762789

Muscular Dystrophies

A muscle disorder in which there is slow but progressive degeneration of muscle fibres. Different forms of muscular dystrophy are classified according to the age at which the symptoms appear and the way in which it is inherited.

DUCHENNE MUSCULAR DYSTROPHY (DMD)

Onset is in early childhood, with progressive muscle weakness. Affected children are chairbound by the age of 12 and usually die in their teenage years. Below average intelligence in 25 per cent of affected boys. About 1 in 3,000 males are affected.

> X-linked recessive inheritance with symptoms in 3 per cent of female carriers. Carrier detection.
> Prenatal diagnosis by fetal sexing and gene tracking or by direct demonstration of the responsible deletion in CVS samples.

BECKER MUSCULAR DYSTROPHY

A less severe, more uncommon form of MD in which muscle weakness begins later in childhood than DMD and progresses more slowly. Incidence is 1 in 20,000 males.

> X-linked recessive inheritance.
> Prenatal diagnosis as for DMD.

MYOTONIC DYSTROPHY

This form affects muscles of the hands and feet. Muscles contract strongly but do not relax easily. Associated with cataracts in middle age, mental retardation and hormonal problems. Affects 1 in 20,000.

> Autosomal dominant. Carrier detection.
> Prenatal diagnosis via CVS or amniocentesis.
> Support group: Muscular Dystrophy Group, 7–11
> Prescott Place, London SW4 6BS 071-720 8055

NEUROFIBROMATOSIS (Café au Lait Syndrome)

Characteristic 'café au lait'-coloured patches on skin before puberty, thereafter neurofibromas develop on the skin and elsewhere on the body. (These are soft growths of fibrous tissue that grow from nerves.) Incidence is about 1 in 4,500. About 25 per cent of those affected will have additional complications which may include mental retardation and scoliosis of the spine.

> Autosomal dominant but 50 per cent of cases due to
> new mutations.
> Prenatal diagnosis via CVS or amniocentesis using gene
> tracking.
> Support group: Link, the Neurofibromatosis Society,
> 120 London Road, Kingston upon Thames, Surrey
> KT2 6QJ 081-547 1636

OSTEOGENESIS IMPERFECTA (Brittle Bones Disease)

There are several types of this condition. Type II is fatal because there are multiple bone fractures at birth. Other types can lead to recurrent fractures. Combined incidence 1 in 20,000.

> Type I is autosomal dominant. Type II does not follow
> a simple inheritance pattern. Type II detectable using
> ultrasound.
> Prenatal diagnosis for Type I via amniocentesis or CVS.

Support group: Brittle Bone Society, 112 City Road,
Dundee DD2 2PW 0382-817771

PHENYLKETONURIA (PKU)

A disorder caused by an enzyme deficiency affecting 1 in
10,000 babies (1 in 7,500 in Scotland) which is usually detected
in newborn babies through the routine Guthrie (heel pinprick)
test. If detected, a childhood diet low in the amino acid
phenylalanine will assure normal development and lifespan.
Diet must be reintroduced during pregnancy as otherwise
there is a risk for the baby of mental retardation and
malformation.

Autosomal recessive. Carrier detection.
Prenatal diagnosis using DNA analysis via
amniocentesis and CVS.
Support group: The National Society for PKU,
7 Southfield Close, Willen, Milton Keynes,
Bucks MK15 9LL 0908-691653

RETINOBLASTOMA

An inherited cancer of the retina (the light–sensitive layer at
the back of the eye) that affects babies and infants. It occurs in
1 in 18,000 babies and can be cured in 90 per cent of cases.
Parents of children with the condition should have their own
eyes tested to check that there are no signs of a spontaneously
regressed retinoblastoma which has gone undetected.

Autosomal dominant (familial cases) but also sporadic
cases.
Presymptomatic diagnosis. Prenatal diagnosis via DNA
analysis using amniocentesis or CVS.
Retinablastoma Society, Moorfield's Eye Hospital, City
Road, London EC1V 2PD
Retinablastoma Society, Academic Department of

Paediatric Oncology, St Bartholomew's Hospital, West Smithfield, London EC1A 7BE 071-600 3309 (Wednesdays only)

SICKLE-CELL DISEASE

A disease in which the red cells of affected people contain an abnormal type of red blood pigment, haemoglobin S. As blood cells reach areas which contain less oxygen such as capillaries, the pigment crystallizes, distorting the red cells into a sickle shape. This sickle shape makes the red blood cells more fragile and easily destroyed, resulting in anaemia. Also, because of their shape, they cannot pass easily through blood vessels. They may then stick in the narrower vessels, restricting blood supply to various organs and causing sickle-cell crises. Sickle-cell anaemia will only occur in individuals who have inherited the gene for haemoglobin S from both parents. If haemoglobin S is inherited from just one parent, an individual will have sickle-cell trait and be free of symptoms. Carrier identification is carried out as much as possible in at-risk populations. Each individual should be given a card showing whether carrier testing is positive or negative. He or she should be counselled as to what these results mean and should be given the name of a support group for further information as required. Incidence in the UK is about 1 in 100 black people of West African origin and 1 in 200 in people of West Indian origin. As many as 1 in 10 blacks in Britain will have sickle-cell trait. In Nigeria, about 1 in 4 people have sickle-cell trait.

Autosomal recessive. Carrier testing.
Prenatal diagnosis via DNA analysis (CVS or amniocentesis) or by direct examination of the baby's blood in second trimester (cordocentesis).
Support group: The Sickle Cell Society, 54 Station Road, London NW10 4UA 081-961 7795/8346

TAY-SACHS DISEASE

A rare but fatal progressive neurological disease which affects 1 in 3,600 Ashkenazi Jews, with 1 in 30 being a carrier.
> Autosomal recessive. Carrier testing.
> Prenatal diagnosis by assay of enzyme in either amniotic or chorionic villi cells obtained by amniocentesis or CVS.
> Support group: British Tay-Sachs Foundation, Jewish Care, 221 Golders Green Road, NW11 9DQ
> 081-458 3282

THALASSAEMIA

This is a form of anaemia which particularly affects people of Mediterranean and Far Eastern origin. It is caused by a disturbance in the body's manufacture of haemoglobin, the red pigment of blood. Haemoglobin contains two pairs of globins (protein chains) known as the alpha and beta chains. In thalassaemias, synthesis of one of these chains is reduced, causing an imbalance between the different chains in much of the haemoglobin that is produced. There are two main types of thalassaemia, caused by a large number of different mutations in the alpha and beta globin genes. In alpha thalassaemia Type 1, in which there are no alpha globin genes, the lack of normal globin chains is incompatible with life, and an affected baby will die within a few hours of birth. There are several lesser degrees of alpha thalassaemia, depending on exactly which alpha globin genes have been inherited, including one which causes chronic anaemia. About 8 per cent of Thais are carriers of alpha thalassaemia 2.

The inheritance of two severe beta globin gene mutations causes thalassaemia major. This is a chronic type of anaemia which has to be treated with repeated blood transfusions as otherwise growth is affected and death would occur in early childhood. Iron overloading, caused by the transfusions, may cause additional problems such as liver cirrhosis, heart failure and diabetes. Daily treatment with an iron chelating agent (Desferal) then becomes essential. Inheritance of only one severe mutation causes less severe disease – so-called thalassaemia minor. Carrier frequency is 1 in 6 in Cypriots, 1 in 14 in Greeks and 1 in 50 in Italians.

The haemoglobin disorders (sickle-cell disease and thalassaemia and its variants) are the commonest genetic disease in inner city areas (with an incidence of 1 per 1,000 in inner London). Bone marrow transplantation from a compatible sibling is an increasingly popular and successful form of treatment for severe forms of these disorders. The haemoglobinopathies are very varied in their precise genetics and most samples are sent to the NHS Haemoglobinopathy Reference Centre at the John Radcliffe Hospital, Oxford.

> *Alpha thalassaemia.* Autosomal recessive. Carrier detection not possible but prenatal diagnosis using DNA analysis via amniocentesis or CVS.
> *Beta thalassaemia.* Autosomal recessive. Very diverse (over 90 mutations of the beta globin gene have been described). Carrier detection with simple blood test. Prenatal diagnosis by DNA analysis via CVS looking for exact mutation if this is known. Alternatively, diagnosis of fetal blood sample obtained by cordocentesis.
> Support group: The UK Thalassaemia Society, 107 Nightingale Lane, London N8 7QY 081-348 0437

TUBEROUS SCLEROSIS

A disorder affecting the skin and the brain. An acne-like rash on the face and other skin problems may be accompanied by epilepsy (in 90 per cent of cases) and mental retardation (60 per cent). A small number (6 per cent) of individuals develop brain tumours. Incidence is 1 in 10,000 births.

Autosomal dominant but 60 per cent of cases are new mutations.
Prenatal diagnosis not possible as yet.
Support group: Tuberous Sclerosis Association, Little Barnsley Farm, Catshill, Bromsgrove, Worcs B61 0NQ
0527-71898

CONGENITAL MALFORMATIONS

A malformation is an error of normal development. All malformations are therefore congenital – that is, present at birth – although some may not be diagnosed until later, especially if they involve internal organs. The cause of 60 per cent of such malformations is unknown. About 3 per cent are associated with maternal illness (such as congenital heart disease in children of diabetic mothers) but genetic conditions account for at least one-third of congenital malformations.

CONGENITAL HEART MALFORMATIONS

Abnormalities of the heart represent the commonest type of congenital malformation with an incidence of 8 in every 1,000 births. If a couple have an affected child, their chances of having another with the same problem are not high. A large number of heart problems have been described, with a ventricular septal defect (hole in the heart) being the most common.

The symptoms of congenital heart disease arise from either not enough or too much blood being sent to either the body or the lungs. Specific defects in heart structure can also mean that blood already depleted in oxygen is pumped to the body instead of to the lungs for oxygenation – this is called 'shunting'. Symptoms including cyanosis (blueness) and breathlessness may occur at any time, over a wide variety of ages, depending on the type of problem. Thus it is possible that a heart problem may not be recognized until adulthood. Surgical correction is becoming more and more successful in an ever greater number of different types of heart problem, although some, such as hypoplastic left heart syndrome (in which the left side of the heart is severely underdeveloped), can only be treated by performing a heart transplant.

> Prenatal diagnosis initially with ultrasound and then with detailed fetal echocardiography at 18–20 weeks at a regional referral centre (see ultrasound, page 87).
> Support group: The Children's Heart Support Federation, 17 Cote Lane, Mossley, Lancs OL5 9DF 0457-833585

Central nervous system

Abnormalities of the central nervous system form the second largest group of congenital malformations. Included among these are macrocephaly (an unusually large head), microcephaly (an abnormally small head), and the neural tube defects, anencephaly and spina bifida.

ANENCEPHALY

The neural tube is the nerve tissue in the embryo that develops into the spinal cord and brain. In anencephaly, defective development of the neural tube results in part of the brain and the cranial vault (the top of the skull) being absent. Incidence is about 16 in every 1,000 conceptions, although only about a third of these pregnancies would normally continue to term, a large number ending as miscarriages. Stillbirth or neonatal death (usually within hours) is inevitable.

The incidence of neural tube defects varies considerably, both worldwide and within different parts of the same country. In the UK, about 3 in every 1,000 babies are affected at birth in London and the South East, rising to 5 in every 1,000 in Glasgow, 7 in every 1,000 in South Wales and 8.6 in every 1,000 in Belfast. There is an increased frequency in lower social classes and with winter-born children. The incidence has fallen quite considerably over the last ten years and this fact seems to be independent of termination of affected pregnancies. Evidence favours the cause of neural tube defects as being multifactorial, i.e. having inherited and environmental components. Folic acid, the nutrient found in green leafy vegetables, is known to be an important factor.

In the UK the recurrence risk after an affected child is 1 in 30. If a second-degree relative has an NTD, the risk is 1 in 70 and for a third-degree relative it is 1 in 150 (see page 133). However, recurrence can be reduced by over 70 per cent if women at risk take 400 microgrammes daily supplement of folic acid both before getting pregnant and in the first three months of pregnancy.

> Prenatal screening using MSAFP and triple test (picks up 90 per cent of anencephalics), diagnosis with ultrasound (100 per cent accuracy).

SPINA BIFIDA

In this neural tube defect, there is an abnormality of development further down the neural tube, resulting in the failure of one or more vertebrae to develop completely, leaving part of the spinal cord exposed. Spina bifida can occur anywhere on the spine, although it is most common in the lumbar area. At birth, the malformation may be closed over by skin (closed lesion) or it may be open. Open spina bifida causes the formation of a sac on the baby's back which contains part of the spinal cord (meningo-myelocele). Depending on its site, a baby may be severely handicapped with partial or complete paralysis in all areas below the level of the defect. Hip dislocation and other leg deformities are common. Paralysis of the bladder and anus leads to incontinence, kidney and bladder problems. Intelligence is not usually affected by spina bifida unless there is a complication as a result of hydrocephalus.

With open lesions corrective surgery within 24 hours is necessary as without surgery only 20 per cent of affected individuals survive to two years of age. After surgery 40 per cent survive to seven years but only 1 per cent are free of handicap. In contrast, 60 per cent of babies with closed lesions survive to five years of age and 30 per cent are free of handicap.

The incidence of neural tube defects and recurrence rates are described under anencephaly. Vitamin supplementation with folate appropriate in next pregnancy.

> Prenatal screening by AFP. Recording of abnormally high level followed by amniocentesis to measure AFP level in amniotic fluid and ultrasound. Also triple test (picks up four out of every five cases of spina bifida). Abnormal result followed by detailed ultrasound scanning. Also ultrasound scanning alone but detection of closed lesions is difficult.
>
> Support group: Association for Spina Bifida and Hydrocephalus (ASBAH), ASBAH House, 42 Park Road, Peterborough, Cambs PE1 2UQ 0733-555988

HYDROCEPHALUS

Better known as water on the brain, this condition occurs when the fluid that cushions and protects the spinal cord accumulates and cannot be reabsorbed into the bloodstream. The excess fluid can cause pressure on the brain and skull and increase head size. It may be secondary to a neural tube defect or the result of infection. It may also be one diagnostic sign of a wider chromosomal problem. With early diagnosis and treatment of isolated hydrocephalus, physical and mental development can be expected to be normal. Treatment can be carried out in utero when a hollow plastic tube called a shunt is inserted into the head under ultrasound guidance, to drain the fluid. However, this will not reverse any effects that have already occurred.

> Prenatal diagnosis by serial measurements of head using ultrasound.
>
> Support group: ASBAH (see under spina bifida)

Abnormalities of the gastrointestinal tract

CLEFT LIP OR PALATE

Cleft lip is a vertical split in the upper lip. Contrary to popular belief, cleft lip is usually off centre. It may be a small notch or extend up to the nose. The upper gum may also be cleft. A cleft palate is a gap in the palate (the roof of the mouth). Depending on its size, the cleft causes the mouth to be in direct contact with the nasal cavity. Cleft lip may occur by itself or with cleft palate, with four out of every nine affected babies having both cleft lip and palate. A degree of deafness may also be associated with cleft palate. Cleft lip and/or palate occurs in 1 in every 1,000 births. Inheritance of these conditions is complex and may be multifactorial although they may also be a feature of over 150 single gene disorders or chromosome abnormalities. Surgery is now very successful in the majority of cases.

> Prenatal diagnosis by ultrasound scanning.
>
> Support group: CLAPA, 1 Eastwood Gardens, Kenton, Newcastle NE3 3DQ 091-285 9396

OESOPHAGEAL ATRESIA

A condition affecting 1 in 3,000 births in which there is an absence of a section of the oesophagus (the tube that carries food to the stomach). Urgent surgical repair is necessary.

> Prenatal diagnosis: ultrasound.

Abnormalities of the abdominal wall

Conditions occurring in 1 in 6,000 pregnancies in which part of the intestines protrude through the navel. In exomphalos, only one or two loops of intestines may be exposed or, in severe cases, most of the abdominal organs. Chromosome abnormalities are also found in 30 per cent of cases. Other conditions of this sort include gastroschisis. Surgical repair can be successful depending on extent of problem.

> Prenatal diagnosis: primarily ultrasound, although such defects often cause an elevation in maternal AFP levels, leading to a positive AFP test.
> Support group: NASPCS (see under obstructive uropathy)

Abnormalities of the kidneys and urinary tract

About 4 in every 1,000 babies will have a defect of the kidneys or urinary tract. Unfortunately many such abnormalities cannot be picked up until relatively late in pregnancy (30 weeks plus). Because the kidneys recycle the amniotic fluid (babies drink the fluid and then pee it into the amniotic cavity), the first sign of these conditions may be a very small amount of amniotic fluid (oligohydramnios).

BILATERAL RENAL AGENESIS

Absence of the kidneys. Neonatal death is invariable. Incidence is about 1 in 3,000 births.

> Prenatal diagnosis: ultrasound at early stage in pregnancy.

OBSTRUCTIVE UROPATHY

A blockage of the ureters, more commonly affecting boys than girls and resulting in oligohydramnios. The prognosis depends on the severity of the obstruction and whether it is associated with additional abnormalities. Surgery in utero has proved successful in a number of cases.

> Prenatal diagnosis: ultrasound but usually later in pregnancy.
> Support group: NASPCS, 51 Anderson Drive, Valley View Park, Darvel, Ayrshire KA17 0DE (also covers intestinal conditions). Also National Federation of Kidney Patients' Associations, 6 Stanley Street, Worksop, Notts S81 7HX 0909-487795

Abnormalities of the limbs

CLUB FOOT (TALIPES)

A defect in which the foot is twisted out of shape or position. Although there may be a genetic factor in some cases, many cases of club foot arise because of compression of the feet by the mother's womb during late pregnancy. It can also occur as a result of oligohydramnios. The condition can be very successfully treated with physiotherapy or occasionally with surgery.

> Prenatal diagnosis sometimes possible by ultrasound.

CHROMOSOMAL DISORDERS

Chromosome disorders include all conditions associated with visible changes of the chromosomes of which there should be 46 (22 pairs of non-sex chromosomes (autosomes) together with a pair of sex chromosomes). In general autosomal abnormalities tend to be more severe than sex chromosome ones and deletions tend to be more severe than duplications.

TRISOMY 21 (Down's syndrome, Mongolism)

The commonest chromosome abnormality occurring in 1 in 700 births. The incidence at conception is far greater but more than 60 per cent of these babies are spontaneously miscarried and 20 per cent stillborn. Incidence increases with maternal age. Arises because there are 47 chromosomes, including one extra No. 21 chromosome. Defective egg formation is more likely to be the cause than abnormal sperm formation (80 per cent to 20 per cent). In 3 per cent of cases, the cause is another chromosome abnormality, a translocation (see glossary) in either parent and this may be an inherited condition. Learning difficulties may be mild to severe. More and more of these children are making the most of their capabilities with sympathetic and constant educational and environmental stimulation. Puberty is often delayed and incomplete with adult height reaching about 150 cm. Presenile dementia commonly occurs after about 40 years of age. About 1 per cent of individuals exhibit mosaicism, having some cells that are normal and some that show Trisomy 21. Such individuals tend to be much less severely affected than in the full syndrome. Risk of recurrence of Trisomy 21 is low (1 per cent), although the age-specific risk needs to be added to this figure if mothers are over 35.

Prenatal diagnosis: screening by triple test (detects 60 per cent of affected babies), karyotyping following

CVS or amniocentesis, increasing use of ultrasound looking for folds of skin around the neck (nuchal folds) and other signs (from 11 weeks). Confirmation by karyotyping usually after cordocentesis.

Support group: Down's Syndrome Association, 155 Mitcham Road, London SW17 9PG 081 682 4001

47, XXY (Klinefelter's syndrome)

Overall birth incidence is 1 per 1,000 males with increased risk with maternal age. It results in poorly developed secondary sexual characteristics. Affected individuals tend to be tall. Infertility is invariable. Severe retardation is uncommon but there is usually some reduction in verbal and mental skills.

Support group: Klinefelter's Syndrome Association, 56 Little Yeldham Road, Little Yeldham, Nr Halstead, Essex 0787-237460

47, XXX

Overall birth incidence is 1 per 1,000 females with a maternal age effect. Individuals are clinically normal but 25 per cent may be mildly mentally retarded.

45, X (Turner's syndrome)

Overall birth incidence is 1 in 5,000 females with the frequency at conception being much higher. Individuals are of normal intelligence and lifespan, but of short stature. Failure of secondary sexual development will result in infertility although occasionally periods may occur and a pregnancy may be possible. Growth hormone may help with a girl's final height. Male Turner's syndrome is the name sometimes given to Noonan syndrome. Although its characteristics are similar (short stature, delayed puberty), they do not share the same cause. Noonan's, which can occur in both males and females, is caused by an autosomal dominant genetic trait.

TRISOMY 18 (Edward's syndrome)

Incidence of this disorder, in which there is an extra chromosome No. 18, is 1 per 3,000 births, with a maternal age effect. There is an excess of affected females but this probably reflects the fact that more boys with this condition are lost as miscarriages. There are multiple abnormalities and 30 per cent die within the first month. For those surviving beyond a year (10 per cent), there is profound developmental delay.

TRISOMY 13 (Patau syndrome)

The incidence of this chromosomal abnormality is 1 in 5,000 births with a maternal age effect. There are multiple malformations including cleft palate and heart disease with only 10 per cent surviving beyond the first year.

> Prenatal diagnosis for all the above conditions is by karyotyping following CVS, amniocentesis or cordocentesis. In addition, physical markers of the conditions involving multiple malformation may be picked up as a result of routine scanning.

FRAGILE X

X-linked mental retardation affects 1 in every 1,000 male births and is the most common cause of moderate and severe mental retardation after Down's syndrome. In addition to mental retardation, affected males may be tall and physically strong with a prominent nose and jaw. The cause is an inherited defect of the X chromosome, the so-called fragile site. This may be seen in up to 60 per cent of cells of affected individuals and may also be seen in a small percentage of cells

from a female carrier who will be unaffected. About a third of
female carriers may show some form of mental retardation.
Prenatal diagnosis would be indicated only where there was a
family history.

> X-linked. Counselling as for an X-linked recessive trait.
> Normal males may transmit the condition to their
> daughters and thence to their grandsons. Carrier
> testing may be possible.
>
> Prenatal diagnosis via a combination of fetal sexing,
> cytogenic analysis and application of linked DNA
> markers following CVS or amniocentesis. Fetal blood
> may also be required for confirmation.
>
> Support group:
> Fragile X Society
> 53 Winchelsea Lane, Hastings
> E. Sussex TN35 4LG
> 0424 813 147

Fetal Medicine Centres in Britain

Aberdeen: Dr M. Hall, Aberdeen Maternity Hospital

Birmingham: Professor M. Whittle, Birmingham Maternity Hospital, Edgbaston

Glasgow: Dr J. Kingdom, Queen Mother's Hospital

Leeds: Professor R. Lilford, St James's University Hospital

London: Professor N. M. Fisk, Queen Charlotte's Maternity Hospital/Hammersmith Hospital
Professor K. Nicolaides, Harris Birthright Centre, King's College Hospital
Professor C. Rodeck, University College Hospital

Manchester: Mr M. Maresh, St Mary's Hospital

Newcastle: Professor T. Lind, Princess Mary Maternity Hospital

Nottingham: Professor D. K. James, City and University Hospitals

Clinical Genetic Centres

ENGLAND

East Anglia Regional Genetic Centre
Regional Genetic Advisory Service, Addenbrooke's Hospital, Hills Road, Cambridge CB2 2QQ

Mersey Regional Genetic Centre
Genetic Advisory Clinic, Maternity Wing, Countess of Chester Hospital, Liverpool Road, Chester CH1 2BA

North East Thames Regional Genetic Centres
Genetic Clinic, Institute of Child Health, The Hospital for Sick Children, Great Ormond Street, London WC1N 3JH

Royal Free Hospital, Pond Street, London NW3 2QG

University College Hospital, Gower Street, London WC1E 6AU

Specialist clinics Hereditary bleeding disorders: Royal Free Hospital, Pond Street, London NW3 2QG

Inherited metabolic disorders: The Hospital for Sick Children, Great Ormond Street London WC1N 3JH

Neurological disorders: The National Hospital for Nervous Diseases, Queen Square, London WC1N 3BG

Ophthalmic disorders: Moorfields Eye Hospital, City Road, London EC1V 2PD

Thalassaemia and sickle-cell disease: University College Hospital, Gower Street, London WC1E 6AU

North West Thames Regional Genetic Centre

The Kennedy Galton Centre, Northwick Park Hospital, Watford Road, Harrow, Middlesex HA1 3UJ

Specialist clinics Dysmorphology: Kennedy Galton Centre, Harperbury Hospital, Harper Lane, Radlett, Herts WD7 9HQ

Neuromuscular disorders: Department of Paediatrics, Hammersmith Hospital, Ducane Road, London W12 0HS

Prenatal diagnosis: Queen Charlotte's Maternity Hospital, Goldhawk Road, London W6 0XG

Sickle-cell disease: The Sickle Cell Centre, Willesden Hospital, Harlesden Lane, London NW10 3RY

North Western Regional Genetic Centres

Department of Clinical Genetics, Royal Manchester Children's Hospital, Pendlebury, Manchester M27 1HA

University Department of Medical Genetics, St Mary's Hospital, Hathersage Road, Manchester M13 0JH

Willinck Biochemical Genetics Laboratory, Royal Manchester Children's Hospital, Pendlebury, Manchester M27 1HA

Northern Regional Genetic Centre

Regional Genetics Advisory Service, University Department of Human Genetics, 19 Claremont Place, Newcastle Upon Tyne NE2 4AA

Oxford Regional Genetic Centre

Department of Medical Genetics, Old Road,
Headington, Oxford OX3 7LE

South East Thames Regional Genetic Centre

Paediatric Research Unit, The Prince Philip Research
Laboratories, Guy's Hospital Medical School, Guy's
Tower, London Bridge SE1 9RT

Specialist clinic   Inherited red cell and coagulation disorders:
Department of Haematological Medicine, King's
College School of Medicine and Dentistry, King's
College London, Bessemer Road London SE5 9PJ

South West Thames Regional Genetic Centre

St George's Hospital, Blackshaw Road, London
SW17 0QT

South Western Regional Genetic Centre

Scott Hospital, Beacon Park Road, Plymouth, Devon
PL2 2PQ

Trent Regional Genetic Centres

Centre for Human Genetics (Sub-department of
Medical Genetics), Langhill, 117 Manchester Road,
Sheffield S10 5ND

The City Hospital, Hucknall Road, Nottingham
NG5 1PD

Genetic Clinic, Leicester Royal Infirmary, Leicester
LE1 5WW

Wessex Regional Genetic Centre

Genetic Clinic, Southampton General Hospital,
Tremona Road, Shirley, Southampton SO9 4XY

West Midlands Regional Genetic Centres

East Birmingham Hospital, Birmingham B9 5ST

Infant Development Unit, Birmingham Maternity
Hospital, Edgbaston, Birmingham B15 2TG

Yorkshire Regional Genetic Centre
Genetic Clinic, Clarendon Wing, Leeds General
Infirmary, Belmont Grove, Leeds LS2 9NS

NORTHERN IRELAND

Northern Ireland Regional Genetic Centre
Department of Medical Genetics, Institute of Clinical
Science, Grosvenor Road, Belfast BT12 6BJ

SCOTLAND

Grampian Regional Genetic Centre
Genetics Clinic, Royal Aberdeen Children's Hospital,
Cornhill Road, Aberdeen AB9 2ZD

Highland Regional Genetic Centre
Paediatric Unit, Raigmore Hospital, Inverness IV2 3UJ

Greater Glasgow Regional Genetic Centre
West of Scotland Regional Genetic Service, Duncan
Guthrie Institute of Medical Genetics, Royal Hospital
for Sick Children, Yorkhill, Glasgow G3 8SJ

Lothian Regional Genetic Centre
Genetic Clinic, Human Genetics Unit, Department of
Medicine, Western General Hospital, Crewe Road,
Edinburgh EH4 2XU

Tayside Regional Genetic Centre
Perth Royal Infirmary, Taymount Terrace, Perth
PH1 1NX

WALES

Wales Regional Genetic Centres

Child Health Laboratories, Welsh National School of
Medicine, Heath Park, Cardiff CF4 4XN

Wales Medical Genetics Clinic, Regional Genetic
Centre, Welsh National School of Medicine, Heath
Park, Cardiff CF4 4XN

General Information Sources

BIRTHRIGHT

The appeal arm of the Royal College of Obstetricians and Gynaecologists. Fundraises for research into problems affecting the health of both women and their babies. Has a special interest in prenatal diagnosis.

> 27 Sussex Place, Regent's Park, London NW1
> 071-723 9296

BRITISH EPILEPSY ASSOCIATION

> Epilepsy Help-line, Anstey House, 40 Hanover Square,
> Leeds LS3 1BE 0305-089599

BRITISH PREGNANCY ADVISORY SERVICE (BPAS)

This organization offers information, counselling and advice on contraception, pregnancy and abortion.

> Head Office Austy Manor Wooten Wawen, Solihull,
> West Midlands B95 6BX 0564-793225

CAF CONTACT-A-FAMILY

Offers advice, support and information to families with children who have any type of disability or special need. Also offers support in setting up and running self-help groups. Holds a central register of conditions and support groups. A national helpline available run by parent advisers:

> 071-222 2695

CARE

This group concentrates on the problems faced by couples in Scotland who decide to terminate a pregnancy where their unborn child has genetic disease or a severe abnormality.

36 Canmore Place, Nether Robertland, Stewarton, Kilmarnock, Ayreshire KA3 5PS 0560-83310

GIG – GENETIC INTEREST GROUP

An umbrella group of voluntary organizations concerned with genetic disorders. Aims to increase public awareness and lobby for improvements and also provides a resources and advice centre for both professionals and people affected.

c/o Institute of Molecular Medicine, John Radcliffe Hospital, Oxford OX3 9DU Helpline: 0865-744002

LET'S FACE IT

Support group for people with facial disfigurements.

10 Wood End, Crowthorne, Berks RG11 6DG 0344-774405

LIFE

188 Warwick Street, Leamington Spa, Warks 0926-311667

MENCAP (ROYAL SOCIETY FOR MENTALLY HANDICAPPED CHILDREN AND ADULTS)

The largest national organization concerned with handicapped people and their families. Local offices and societies raise money and offer a wide range of services to the handicapped and their families.

123 Golden Lane, London EC1Y 0RT 071-253 9433

THE MISCARRIAGE ASSOCIATION

Provides help, support and information to women and their families.

18 Stoneybrook Close, West Bretton, Wakefield, W. Yorks 092-485 515

THE NATIONAL CHILDBIRTH TRUST

Promotes antenatal preparation with a national network of groups offering classes for the pregnant woman and her partner.

Alexandra House, Oldham Terrace, Acton, London
W3 6NH 081-992 8637

RESEARCH TRUST FOR METABOLIC DISEASES IN CHILDREN

This includes a range of 1,300 life-threatening conditions where a catalyst or enzyme is either missing or does not function properly, affecting the chemical balance within the body. The trust offers information and support to families and has a network of parent support groups.

Golden Gates Lodge, Weston Road, Crewe, Cheshire
CW1 1XN 0270-250221

SANDS (STILLBIRTH AND NEONATAL DEATH SOCIETY)

A national self-help network of parents offering support and information. Particularly helpful about provisions for funerals etc.

28 Portland Place, London W1 071-436 5881

SATFA (SUPPORT AFTER TERMINATION FOR ABNORMALITY)

For those parents facing a prenatal diagnosis of fetal abnormality, this group offers information, support and counselling.

29–30 Soho Square, London W1V 6JB 071-439 6124

SCOLIOSIS ASSOCIATION

2 Iverbury Court, 323-327 Latimer Road, London W10
6RA 081-964 5343

SENSE (THE NATIONAL DEAF BLIND AND RUBELLA ASSOCIATION)

The organization offers support, advice and information, advocacy if necessary and help with welfare benefits.

311 Gray's Inn Road, London WC1X 8PT
071-278 1005

SOCIETY FOR THE PROTECTION OF THE UNBORN CHILD
7 Tufton Street London SW1P 3QN 071-222 5845

TOXOPLASMOSIS TRUST
61–71 Collier Street London N1 9BE 071–713 0663

TWINS AND MULTIPLE BIRTHS ASSOCIATION
Practical support and advice for parents with twins, triplets or more.

PO Box 30, Little Sutton, South Wirral L66 1TH
051 348 0020

VOLUNTARY COUNCIL FOR HANDICAPPED CHILDREN
An advisory body on all aspects of childhood disability providing information for parents and professionals.

National Children's Bureau, 8 Wakley Street, London
EC1U 7QE 071-278 9441

Glossary

ALLELE The alternative form of a gene or DNA sequence occurring at the same spot on the other chromosome of a chromosome pair. Any gene may have several different alleles.

ANEUPLOIDY A condition in which there are either extra chromosomes (such as Down's syndrome, 47 chromosomes), or missing chromosomes (Turner's syndrome, 45 chromosomes) in each cell.

AUTOSOME Any chromosome other than the sex chromosomes, i.e. chromosomes Nos 1–22 in human beings. An autosomal genetic disease will affect boys and girls equally. **Autosomal dominant** is explained in detail on page 13. An individual possessing an autosomal dominant gene will have characteristics of a particular disorder. There is a 50 per cent chance of a child being affected in every pregnancy. **Autosomal recessive** is explained in detail on page 11. An individual carrying an autosomal recessive gene will not be affected by it themselves but when two carriers of this gene have children, there is a 1 in 4 chance of an affected child in every pregnancy.

CARRIER An individual who carries an abnormal gene for a disorder without being affected by it.

CHROMATID The two halves into which a chromosome is longitudinally divided at mitosis and meiosis.

CHROMOSOMES The rod-like structures present in the central portion (nucleus) of all cells (with a few exceptions such as some red blood cells). They store genetic information in the form of a long, unbroken chemical chain which is then tightly coiled. The chemical is called DNA (qv). Humans have 23 pairs of chromosomes in each cell, except in sperm and egg which have only 23 single chromosomes. Chromosomes can be seen with the aid of a high-powered microscope. They are not visible to the naked eye.

CONGENITAL   A condition present at birth.

DELETION The absence of genetic material on a chromosome.

DIPLOID   The normal number of chromosomes in all cells, i.e. 23 pairs, except those of sperm and egg which are said to contain the haploid number, i.e. 23 single chromosomes.

DISCORDANCE   A genetic trait (qv) which is apparent in only one of a pair of twins.

DISOMY, UNIPARENTAL   The inheritance of both members of a pair of chromosomes from one parent (instead of having one from each), with the loss of the corresponding pair from the other parent. Uniparental disomy is a cause of miscarriage and also may result in poor growth of the baby during pregnancy.

DIZYGOTIC   Where two eggs have been fertilized giving rise to non-identical twins.

DNA   The chemical from which chromosomes are made. DNA stands for deoxyribonucleic acid.

DNA PROBE   A bit like a sniffer dog trained to find a single thing, a DNA probe is a radioactive piece of DNA that will link up only with another piece of DNA that has a complementary sequence of genes. There are lots of DNA probes, each manufactured specifically to find one gene or sequence of genes.

DUPLICATION   Occurs where a chromosome or part of a chromosome is duplicated.

ENZYME   Chemicals in the body which act as catalysts, speeding up the normal processes of the body, particularly those involving the breakdown of food into essential chemicals or the breakdown of toxic by-products in the body.

EXON   Only a small fraction of the total DNA is occupied by specific coding sequences (exons). Each gene may contain non-coding sequences (introns) as well as exons. The introns are spliced out before the gene's information is 'read'. Between genes there are non-coding intergene sequences which seem to act rather like the punctuation or chapter headings in a book.

EXPRESSION   A term used to describe whether a particular gene has affected an individual, e.g. someone may have a red hair gene but have brown hair. If the red hair gene is 'expressed' it simply means that an individual has red hair.

FAMILIAL   Characteristic of some or all members of a family.

GAMETES   Sperm or egg.

GENE   A length of DNA controlling the manufacture of chemicals associated with a particular inherited characteristic.

GENOTYPE   The genetic constitution of an organism. This can be different from the phenotype (qv).

HAPLOID   The normal number of chromosomes in sperm or egg, i.e. 23 single chromosomes in human beings.

HETEROZYGOTE   Someone possessing different variants of the same gene on the same site of each of a pair of chromosomes.

HOMOZYGOTE   Someone possessing identical copies of the same gene on the same site of each of a pair of chromosomes.

INCIDENCE   The rate at which new cases of a particular disorder appear. For disorders present at birth, a figure is usually given per 1,000 or 10,000 births (birth incidence). Note that the prevalence (qv) of a disorder is usually lower than the incidence, because of the reduced life expectancy of individuals with a particular problem.

INVERSION   Occurs where part of a chromosome becomes detached and then reattached, only the other way round, so that a portion of the chromosome reads backwards.

KARYOTYPE   A formal record of the chromosome picture

of an individual in which all the chromosomes of a single cell are displayed in a systematic way. In this way, any abnormal chromosome configuration is easier to identify. Particular attention is paid to the number of chromosomes present, what shape and size they are, how many sex chromosomes are present, etc.

MEIOSIS The process of cell division which results in a cell in which there are only half the number of chromosomes, i.e. 23 singles instead of 23 pairs.

MITOSIS The normal process of cell division which occurs in all cells except those of sperm and egg, and which results in two new cells each with an identical genetic make-up to that of the parent cell.

MONOSOMY The loss of one of a pair of chromosomes e.g. in Turner's syndrome where one X chromosome is lost, resulting in only 45 chromosomes instead of 46. This would be written 45, X.

MOSAICISM Where a genetic abnormality does not occur in all body cells. The proportion of body cells with the abnormality may determine the severity of the disease.

MULTIFACTORIAL A condition which is multifactorial in origin is not caused by a single gene but a series of unrelated genes which not only act together but also interact with the environment. Examples of multifactorial disorders are neural tube defects, for instance, spina bifida and cleft palate.

MUTANT A gene which has undergone change from the normal gene. Mutations occur quite naturally at a rate which can be predicted. For instance, mutation rate for the type of dwarfism known as achondroplasia is about 1 in 100,000, i.e. once in every 100,000 times the normal allele (qv) mutates to give the abnormal dominant gene that causes this condition. In general the rate at which new genes, arising by mutation, are being fed into the population is balanced by the rate at which abnormal genes are being eliminated owing to the lowered reproductive rate of their possessors. This explains why termination of all babies affected by a particular abnormality would not eliminate the abnormality from the population. The mutation rate of all genes can be greatly increased by outside agents. Radio-activity is the best known example but certain chemicals, for instance, mustard gas, greatly speed up the mutation rate. Mutations may not necessarily be passed to the next generation. A blue spot in the eye of a brown-eyed person is an example of so-called somatic mutation.

NON-DISJUNCTION When a chromosome pair fails to separate, usually during formation of sperm and egg, resulting in some cells that have a pair of chromosomes instead of one single chromosome and others that have none.

OBLIGATE CARRIER A family member who, from the pattern of affected individuals within a family and what is known about the way in which a particular disorder is inherited, can be deduced to be a carrier.

PENETRANCE An individual who carries a dominant gene for a disorder can show a variable degree of symptoms from hardly affected to chronically disabled. This is described as the degree of penetrance.

POLYMERASE CHAIN REACTION (PCR) A new laboratory technique in which a very small piece of genetic material is duplicated many, many times. Having more of a particular gene sequence makes it easier to carry out identification tests.

PREVALENCE The proportion of the whole population affected at any one time by a disorder, usually given as a number per 1,000 or 100,000.

PROBAND A term used in genetic counselling to indicate the affected individual who brings a family to the attention of the genetic counsellor.

TRANSLOCATION   Occurs when there is an exchange of genetic material between one chromosome and any other of a different pair. There are several types of translocation. In some families, Down's syndrome is not caused by non-disjunction but as a result of translocation. In these families, the likelihood of another baby affected by Down's is significantly increased above the normal age-dependent risk. *Reciprocal translocations* occur when two chromosomes break and exchange places, in such a way that no genetic material is actually lost. An individual with a so-called balanced translocation may be unaffected by it, but it may have implications for the children of that individual. *Robertsonian translocations* occur when the translocations involve end-to-end fusion of the chromosomes, with a complete loss of the short arms. This will result in a carrier of this type of translocation having only 45 chromosomes. The carrier will be normal but any children may be affected in a number of different ways.

TRIPLOIDY   The presence of a full extra set of chromosomes. This chromosome configuration is usually lethal and would lead to either miscarriage or stillbirth.

TRISOMY   The addition of a complete extra chromosome to a pair as in Down's syndrome where there are three chromosomes No. 21 instead of two.

X-LINKED RECESSIVE   The type of inheritance where the abnormal gene is carried on the X chromosome. Usually girls are carriers of X-linked diseases (haemophilia is probably the best known example) and boys are affected. This is because the male Y chromosome is little and does not carry the compensatory normal gene.

Index